Following the
Great Physician

Following the Great Physician

A Doctor's Guide to Trusting God and Serving Patients

Melissa Khalil, MD

Copyright © 2020 by Melissa Khalil

Following the Great Physician

All rights reserved. This book is protected by the copyright laws of the United States of America. This book may not be copied or reprinted for commercial gain or profit. The use of short quotations or occasional page copying for personal or group study is permitted and encouraged. Permission will be granted upon request from Melissa Khalil.

Although the author has made every effort to ensure that the information in this book was correct at press time, the author and publisher do not assume and hereby disclaim any liability to any party for any loss, damage, or disruption caused by errors or omissions, whether such errors or omissions result from negligence, accident, or any other cause.

The resources in this book are provided for informational purposes only and should not be used to replace the specialized training and professional judgment of a health care or mental health care professional. Neither the author nor the publisher can be held responsible for the use of the information provided within this book. Please always consult a trained professional before making any decision regarding treatment of yourself or others.

Unless otherwise identified, Scripture quotations are taken from the New King James Version®, Copyright © 1982 by Thomas Nelson. Used by permission. All rights reserved. Scripture quotations marked NIV are taken from THE HOLY BIBLE, NEW INTERNATIONAL VERSION®, Copyright © 1973, 1978, 1984, 2011 by Biblica, Inc.® Used by permission. All rights reserved worldwide. Scripture quotations marked TPT are taken from The Passion Translation®, Copyright © 2017, 2018 by Passion & Fire Ministries, Inc. Used by permission. All rights reserved. ThePassionTranslation.com. Scripture quotations marked MSG are taken from THE MESSAGE, Copyright © 1993, 2002, 2018 by

Eugene H. Peterson. Used by permission of NavPress. All rights reserved. Represented by Tyndale House Publishers, Inc. Scripture quotations marked NLT are taken from the Holy Bible, New Living Translation, Copyright © 1996, 2004, 2015 by Tyndale House Foundation. Used by permission of Tyndale House Publishers, Inc., Carol Stream, Illinois 60188. All rights reserved. Any emphasis added to Scripture quotations is the author's own.

Following the Great Physician: A Doctor's Guide to Trusting God and Serving Patients – 1st ed.

Editing and layout by James L Bryson (JamesLBryson@gmail.com)

Cover design by 100 Covers (100covers.com)

ISBN 978-0-5786-2848-6

Endorsements

Have you ever asked yourself, "How can I serve God and at the same time pursue my career?" Have you been struggling with the thought that living your Christian life and pursuing your calling as a Christian is not compatible with living your dream and being at the marketplace or in your job responsibilities? Are you a doctor or a marketplace worker that is struggling to find time for God in your busy routine? Well I think you should read this book!

I have watched Dr. Melissa as her pastor during all the hard years of studying as a medical student, I have seen her struggle, I have encountered her many times of feeling tired. As she went through all these years and looking back, I can say that she is an example to follow. In many ways, Dr. Melissa is a hero in being a winner in reconciling her calling to her studying pursuit. Her great testimony will help you answer most of the questions that any Christian doctor is facing or maybe even any marketplace Christian might be going through.

I have known Dr. Melissa for a long time now (13 years) and I have witnessed the way God has raised her and made her a great minister and a wonderful doctor with good news.

I do recommend this book to be read with the light and guidance of the Holy Spirit and may this testimony find all those that need to hear it and be blessed by it and moreover experience the same blessings that Dr. Melissa Khalil did.

Chady El Aouad
Sr. Pastor at Abundant Life Church & Ministries
Beirut-Lebanon

In this excellent writing, Dr. Melissa Khalil has captured the most essential concepts of faith and God's great desire to use us as His vessels of healing and light to this world. The ultimate partnership of God using mankind is the incredible calling for each one of us. God wants to use all of us to bring His love and His healing power to our world.

There is a story in the Old Testament where a plague moved into Israel and they began to suffer and die. God commanded Moses to make a Brazen Serpent and lift it up on a rock, so that the people could look upon it and be healed. I love how this story relates to physicians' Hippocratic Oath and their emblem of a serpent upon a rod, pointing us all to the cross of Jesus Christ for sickness and also for sin. For all of us, whatever you go through, remember to look to the Cross (ref. Numbers 21:8).

Look to Jesus and be made whole. Thank God for doctors who look to Jesus. God bless you.

Randy Needham
Sr. Pastor at Dwelling Place Church
Houston-Texas

As the daughter of a surgical oncologist, I have had the privilege of observing the tremendous impact of when Faith and Science merge together. When these two streams flow as one, doctors can function at their highest capacity. My father's patients were always extremely grateful that he partnered with the Divine Physician on their behalf. Many received healings and unquestionable interventions. The Lord was the source of not only his outstanding medical achievements, but He was the power and emotional strengthener of his life. He walked trusting in The Lord for his patients and for his own life as well. May you do the same.

This excellent book is written to encourage you in your magnificent journey. It is thorough, straight forward, and beautifully written. Go through it slowly and prayerfully, and don't just read it once! May it forever change your medical practice, and most of all, your life.

Lucie Needham
Pastor at Dwelling Place Church
Houston-Texas

Dedication

For my parents – Never has a moment passed where I couldn't see and feel your unconditional love towards me. You taught me how beautiful life is when helping others. You demonstrated this by your endless support to your children every single day of their lives. Thank you for all the sacrifices you made for us to be where we are today. I pray I will one day be such an outstanding parent to my children. Thank you for guiding me to the lover of my heart, Jesus. I am exceptionally blessed to have both of you in my life. You are my priceless treasure. I love you!

For my brother Cliff – It is not by chance that we love to do the exact same things, without exception, from the smallest activities to becoming doctors. I have always looked up to you as my big brother and my hero. Thank you for always believing in me, encouraging me and sharing my childhood dreams. I pray that this time, we both walk and share this significant calling of becoming Christ-like physicians. I love you!

For every medical student and doctor – You are the hope of the medical field. Thank you for your dedication and great accomplishments. I pray that you find your true callings and experience God's mighty power in you and through you. I also pray that, as we follow the Great Physician, we will cross paths and form a beautiful community of Christ-like doctors.

Table of Contents

Introduction xv
1. Our Responsibilities as Doctors 1
   Offer Our Best 1
   Be Our Best 19
2. My Wilderness Journey 33
3. Completed in Christ 43
   We Are The Patient's Hope 43
   Intercession 49
   Learn From Jesus 57
   What Bothers You Matters 67
4. Trusting God 81
   Fill Your Cup 85
   Study And Work Will Never End 89
   Bitter To Sweet 93
   Take The Burden Of God's Kingdom 98
5. Becoming Successful 105
   God's Love Is Better Than Life 106
   Getting Closer To Jesus 114
   Run Your Own Race 122
   We Are Special 126

6. Work-Life Balance 131
    Rest In God 131
    Rest Is A Gift 138
    Glory To Glory 143
    Peace Through It All 151
    An Ounce Of Prevention 154
Conclusion 157
Acknowledgements 159
About the Author 161
Can You Help? 161

Introduction

Then He called His twelve disciples together and gave them power and authority over all demons, and to cure diseases. He sent them to preach the kingdom of God and to heal the sick.

He received them (the multitudes) and spoke to them about the kingdom of God, and healed those who had need of healing.

Luke 9:1-2, 11

After equipping His disciples with power and authority, Jesus sent them out, commissioning them to proclaim the Kingdom of God and heal the sick. As doctors, we continue that commission. Yet, our calling goes far beyond merely saving lives. It is not enough to make people physically well. We are called to demonstrate and establish God's Kingdom through our lives as doctors.

Two years before graduating from medical school, I was faced with a crisis. *Medicine is getting harder every day and I can't do what I want to, which is to serve God in this journey.*

This was a tragic reckoning. Medicine was everything I wanted to do from early childhood. But since age 15, my heart's longing has been to live for Christ. With the increasing demands of medicine, I felt it was impossible for me to achieve my desire. In the midst of medical student burnout, I decided to quit medicine and go into full-time ministry. As much as I wanted to leave my chosen career, however, the Lord was even more gracious and prevented me from taking that step, which for me, would have been defeat. Through His unfailing mercy, I graduated from medical school. From this process grew the desire to help others in medicine who might be facing similar situations, either in medical school or actual practice.

It is for this reason that I dedicate this book to all medical students and physicians desiring to live for Christ but who may find themselves stressed or broken by the difficulties of a medical career.

I dream of a community of doctors who believe in the mighty name of Jesus and His supernatural healing power as a daily way of living. Jesus is still the Healer, Comforter and Cornerstone. He is the Great Physician, the perfect example to follow.

This book was written through many tears, tests and triumphs as the Holy Spirit ministered to me during my burnout. In those difficult months, I asked God repeatedly why He wanted me to pursue a life in medicine. I could not see any possible way to serve him in this endeavor. Yet as I drew nearer to Jesus, He answered my questions and dealt with the insecurities that had been rending my heart.

My writing began as a healing process for me. Now it is for you and me—the medical community seeking to serve God. Let it be our guide as we enter new seasons of trusting God and serving our patients.

May Jesus give us insights of how He dealt with the sick. May He reveal the authority He has imparted to each of us as believers in Him. May He show us His true desire, which is for us to live successfully and enjoy our lives as Christian medical doctors.

Many blessings,

Melissa

1

Our Responsibilities as Doctors

You shall love your neighbor as yourself.

Mark 12:31

1. OFFER OUR BEST

He walked in the patient's room and yelled: "Everybody out! I don't want any family members or friends in here."

He then turned to the patient—a 75-year-old lady so frail she could barely move—and shouted, "Sit up so I can examine you."

I was appalled. Seeing her weakened state, I rushed to help her. Ignoring her struggles, the doctor approached her with cold indifference in his eyes. His examination was the personification of arrogance. It shattered all my expectations of what an experienced doctor's manner should be. As I followed him on his rounds, the scene repeated itself with every patient.

Questions racked my young mind.

Why is he doing that?

Is he a real doctor or a rogue cowboy from a 1950's western?

How could any doctor be so insensitive?

How long would a patient accept this harsh behavior?

In the proceeding days, I learned that he was an intelligent and skilled physician. But still, what kind of satisfaction did the patient get in return apparent abuse? If I was the patient, I'd have sought a less-skilled doctor than this cold-hearted egotist. This is because the practice of medicine goes far beyond the science of fixing the human body.

"Medicine is a calling, not a job," the saying goes. I couldn't agree more. Unfortunately, many physicians fall in love with the heart of medicine—the biological challenge of healing. Yet because of the profession's difficult journey to acquire and apply medical knowledge and skills on human beings, their hearts grow hard and bitter.

Learning to be compassionate requires that we become humble and highly value others.

Naturally, every physician would like to hear: "You are a great doctor! I am forever grateful for your service." But not every patient appreciates the care being given or the effort behind it. Just as not all doctors are perfect, neither are all patients. Some are ungrateful and rude. We doctors have to learn that illness does not always bring out the best in people.

I have learned to put myself in my patient's shoes. Understanding what is expected of me helps me provide the best care possible. As a patient, I would love for a doctor to treat me as they would treat a member of their family. Indeed, they should treat me even better.

The key is to love our patients as ourselves, as Jesus commanded us to do. We can break this down into key components.

COMPASSION

Patients look for a doctor who is compassionate, who treats them like their own family and friends, the way they would like to be treated. A patient doesn't want to be discriminated against because of finances, education, social standing, race or gender. Instead, a patient desires and deserves a level of compassion as Jesus displayed in scripture.

> *So Jesus had compassion and touched their eyes. And immediately their eyes received sight, and they followed Him.*
>
> Matthew 20:34
>
> *But when He saw the multitudes, He was moved with compassion for them, because they were weary and scattered, like sheep having no shepherd.*
>
> Matthew 9:36
>
> *When the Lord saw her, He had compassion on her and said to her, "Do not weep."*
>
> Luke 7:13

As we see in these verses, Jesus' compassion led Him to heal the sick, raise the dead, and feed the hungry—not only the physically hungry but also the spiritually hungry. Of course, Jesus only did what He saw His Father do.

> *Then Jesus answered and said to them, "Most assuredly, I say to you, the Son can do nothing of Himself, but what He sees the Father do; for whatever He does, the Son also does in like manner."*
>
> John 5:19

Our God is full of compassion. As doctors, we need to look to our Father and do what He does to the best of our abilities.

> *The Lord is gracious and full of compassion, slow to anger and great in mercy.*
>
> Psalm 145:8

Sadly, I know many intelligent doctors who ignore compassion as a necessary skill. Nothing hurts worse than seeing their patients being treated brutally. I often wonder why patients accept such behavior. The physical pain of illness is bad enough. Why would they endure emotional and psychological pain as well? The truth is that for most sick people, the ability to stand up for themselves—especially to someone in authority—is diminished by their ailments.

Let's face it: sickness is difficult to deal with. Whenever I'm ill, my whole world stops, and I feel vulnerable. The last thing I want is to be mistreated or misunderstood by the medical expert I am presenting myself to for help.

Doctors should be compassionate human beings because they work with broken people desperate for good health, bargaining for a few more months of life, seeking a means to walk again, or sometimes just desiring a peaceful death.

> *Therefore, as God's chosen people, holy and dearly loved, clothe yourselves with compassion, kindness, humility, gentleness and patience.*
>
> Colossians 3:12 NIV

Respect

A patient deserves respect from their physician. While modern society in general becomes more self-centered and arrogant, the Lord asks us to clothe ourselves with kindness and humility. Nothing in this world—neither materialistic nor intellectual—gives us the right to disrespect others. We are all brothers and sisters in Christ. We all need each other, and we have a right to the respect of others.

Consider again this powerful message by Jesus.

> *The first of all the commandments is: "Hear, O Israel, the Lord our God, the Lord is one. And you shall love the Lord your God with all your heart, with all your soul, with all your mind, and with all your strength." This is the first commandment. And the second, like it, is this: "You shall love your neighbor as yourself." There is no other commandment greater than these."*
>
> Mark 12:29-31

Jesus said that loving your neighbor as yourself was one of the two most important commandments from the heart of God. It doesn't get any bigger than that.

> *Therefore if there is any consolation in Christ, if any comfort of love, if any fellowship of the Spirit, if any affection and mercy, fulfill my joy by being like-minded, having the same love, being of one accord, of one mind. Let nothing be done through selfish ambition or conceit, but in lowliness of mind let each esteem others better than himself. Let each of you*

> *look out not only for his own interests, but also for the interests of others.*
>
> Philippians 2:1-4

Every doctor should make this passage a personal declaration. Medicine should not be done *through selfish ambition or conceit*, and yet we see it time after time. The solution is in the same verse: *in lowliness of mind let each esteem others better than himself.*

<u>QUALITY TIME</u>

One of the areas of respect is good time management. The patient should be given enough time with the physician to ask questions, express what is on their mind, and even react emotionally if need be.

Now, to a busy doctor, this can be overwhelming when a patient takes an inordinate amount of time. Let us look at how Jesus responded when people followed him from town to town clamoring for his time and attention. This event occurred immediately after John the Baptist was beheaded:

> *When Jesus heard it, He departed from there by boat to a deserted place by Himself. But when the multitudes heard it, they followed*

Him on foot from the cities. And when Jesus went out He saw a great multitude; and He was moved with compassion for them, and healed their sick.

Matthew 14:13-14

It is important to note that John was Jesus' relative. They likely knew each other while growing up. The Old Testament talks about John in Malachi 3:1 as "My messenger, and he will prepare the way before Me." John is referred to in Isaiah 40:3 as "The voice of one crying in the wilderness: 'Prepare the way of the Lord'." Jesus said: "Assuredly, I say to you, among those born of women there has not risen one greater than John the Baptist" (Matthew 11:11).

So clearly John was a mighty man of God and a promise for the people of God. Jesus, who used to spend his days teaching and healing the crowds, now seems deeply saddened by John's death. He is seeking solitude. However, when He sees the crowds following him to the other town and *as sheep without a shepherd*, He has compassion on them and heals their sick.

How amazing would it be if, out of an overflow of love, we would care for patients as the sons and daughters of the Lord Almighty, people desperate for hope. Would this caring motivate us beyond our immediate needs? Would we find new purpose in giving to our patients?

> *You are the salt of the earth… You are the light of the world.*
>
> Matthew 5:13-14

Let us be the salt and light of the world, and let us give our patients our full attention.

In Matthew 14, we saw how Jesus, hurt by the bad news about John, did not complain nor abandon the hurting crowds. Instead, He subordinated His emotions and continued to heal the sick.

In medicine, disciplining my thoughts and emotions is key to fully engaging my attention for the patient's best. Patients have much to say beyond reciting their physical complaints. We, as doctors, should dedicate time to listen to whatever they want to express. The doctor is not just dealing with diseases. We are to treat the patient as a whole person. A doctor has a mission to put others first and serve God in a community of hurting people. This includes listening to them.

Nowadays, we know that many physical diseases are caused by stress and psychological pain. Therefore, taking a comprehensive patient history is key to a correct diagnosis. Modern medicine is not only about lab work, imaging and treatments. A big part of medicine relies on *receiving and analyzing* what the patient has to say.

Notice in this famous passage how Jesus gave his "patient" His full attention. Jesus was on His way to heal the daughter of a synagogue leader when a woman with an ailment touched his cloak.

> *Now a woman, having a flow of blood for twelve years, who had spent all her livelihood on physicians and could not be healed by any, came from behind and touched the border of His garment. And immediately her flow of blood stopped.*
>
> *And Jesus said, "Who touched Me?"*
>
> *When all denied it, Peter and those with him said, "Master, the multitudes throng and press You, and You say, 'Who touched Me?'"*
>
> *But Jesus said, "Somebody touched Me, for I perceived power going out from Me." Now when the woman saw that she was not*

> *hidden, she came trembling; and falling down before Him, she declared to Him in the presence of all the people the reason she had touched Him and how she was healed immediately.*
>
> *And He said to her, "Daughter, be of good cheer; your faith has made you well. Go in peace."*
>
> Luke 8:43-48

Jesus, knowing that power had gone out of Him, stopped everything and waited to see who touched His robe. It was a chaotic scene. "As Jesus was on his way, the crowds almost crushed him" (Luke 8:42 NIV).

Notice too that when He stopped to ask who touched Him, His disciples tried to get Him to ignore it.

> *"When all denied it, Peter and those with him said, "Master, the multitudes throng and press You, and You say, 'Who touched Me?'"*
>
> Luke 8:45

The easy thing was for Jesus to shrug his shoulders, take the advice of His disciples and move on under the momentum of the crowd. However, for Him, that powerful moment was worth His full attention. I believe He knew who had touched Him, but He stopped because He wanted to acknowledge the woman's faith in front of everyone else and for the generations to come.

Notice how Jesus not only provided healing to the woman, but He also paused to bless her spiritually and emotionally.

> *And He said to her, "Daughter, be of good cheer; your faith has made you well. Go in peace."*

Luke 8:48

In the NIV, the words are translated:

> *He said to her, "Daughter, your faith has healed you. Go in peace and be freed from your suffering."*

Mark 5:34

Patients need to feel loved, secure, and cared for. We should be sensitive to every hint the patient might offer to provide them with the best care possible. We are to be the hope for the hopeless.

It starts with our time and attention.

Best Care

It is the right of every patient to be fully informed about treatment options, including recommendations for the best care for their situation. So, what if the best we have is not enough? What if medical treatment fails?

Medicine is much more than a job. If we have given our lives to Christ, we must realize that we were called to be doctors. The Lord Himself called His sons and daughters into this broken world to be the light of the world. How much more should doctors be the hope of hurting patients.

> *His disciples asked him, "Rabbi, who sinned, this man or his parents, that he was born blind?" "Neither this man not his parents sinned," said Jesus, "but this happened so that the works of God might be displayed in him. As long as it is day, we must do the works of him who sent me. Night is coming, when no one can work. While I am in the world, I am the light of the world."*
>
> John 9:2-5 NIV

Jesus said "*we* must do the works of him who sent me." Who is "we"? Well, in Jesus' case, He teamed up with His disciples to do the Father's will. Today, Jesus is the team leader, and He has chosen us for greater works.

> *Most assuredly, I say to you, he who believes in Me, the works that I do he will do also; and greater works than these he will do, because I go to My Father.*
>
> John 14:12

So, let us be the pleasing aroma of Christ that brings hope and healing to the world. Let us clothe ourselves with Christ so that He shines through us, glorifying God through our work. Then we will see Him move mightily just as He promised.

The greatest burden of a patient-physician relationship is that they are entrusting me with their lives. As heavy as this is, however, we as Christians carry an even greater responsibility—the souls of those around us, the people with whom the Lord has entrusted us. Jesus died for you and me so that we could have eternal life in His Holy Presence. My first assignment, therefore, is to bring the gospel to the world and proclaim God's mercy and grace. Medicine is one way to accomplish that assignment.

Indeed, some medical specialties have lighter responsibilities, yet with others, the patient's life is literally in the physician's hands. Whichever is the case, our responsibility is to diagnose, make the best decision, and offer the best treatment. Although it can be overwhelming, God is calling us to trust Him through it all.

We should start our day crying out to the Lord as our only help. He is omniscient and He works on our behalf. If we ask, He is faithful to give us the wisdom we need to care for our patients.

God is the alpha and the omega, the first and the last, the Lord who gives and takes away. As I surrender all to Him, God acknowledges my faithfulness. He completes my work with success. It is the doctor's responsibility to take the best care of the patient, as much as a person can. Yet I must be ready when God calls a patient home. That's when a person leaves this earth and enters the eternal kingdom.

My assignment is to work as for the Lord. But God also calls me to lean back into His arms, resting in the fact that He is my loving Father. When I feel overwhelmed by my responsibilities as a doctor, He wants me to leave all of my cares at the cross.

Consider the song of King David, who carried the responsibility for an entire nation.

> *To You, O Lord, I lift up my soul.*
> *O my God, I trust in You;*
> *Let me not be ashamed;*
> *Let not my enemies triumph over me.*
> *Indeed, let no one who waits on You be ashamed;*
> *Let those be ashamed who deal treacherously without cause.*
> *Show me Your ways, O Lord;*
> *Teach me Your paths.*
> *Lead me in Your truth and teach me,*
> *For You are the God of my salvation;*
> *On You I wait all the day.*
> *Remember, O Lord, Your tender mercies and Your lovingkindnesses,*
> *For they are from of old.*
>
> Psalm 25:1-6

Prayer

The cry of my heart is to know You Lord as my one and only counselor—all day and every day.

> *For unto us a Child is born,*
> *Unto us a Son is given;*
> *And the government will be upon His shoulder.*
> *And His name will be called*
> *Wonderful, Counselor, Mighty God,*
> *Everlasting Father, Prince of Peace.*
>
> Isaiah 9:6

You are the all-knowing God! My knowledge will never be enough, but because of Your unfailing grace, I can boldly say that with You, I am strong.

> *Oh, the depth of the riches both of the wisdom and knowledge of God! How unsearchable are His judgments and His ways past finding out!*
>
> Romans 11:33

> *And He said to me, "My grace is sufficient for you, for My strength is made perfect in weakness."*
>
> 2 Corinthians 12:9

Lord Jesus, You said that if I ask for wisdom, You will give abundantly. I come before You and I ask for wisdom in my work to take the best decisions for my patients. We live on every word You say, and I thank You because all You say is full of life and hope.

2. BE OUR BEST

Most doctors excel in undergraduate school, and when they choose medicine, they think it's going to be the same. At least this is what happened to me. I found out quickly, however, that medical school is nothing like undergraduate school. The crushing weight of the studies, the scant time we get to ourselves, the internships of constant scrutiny, and the twenty-four-hour shifts are all parts of a whirlwind that can consume us.

As doctors, we have high expectations of ourselves. All our lives we have been the smart ones, the gifted, those that people expected much from. No wonder we measure success by high grades, class standing, and our ability to constantly give our best.

Yet when we fail to meet our lofty standards, fear and doubt creep in.

I am not good enough.
I picked the wrong career.
I am not where I am supposed to be.

That's what happened to me. From the time I was five, I was always in the top students of my class. Then I started medical school. The competition was staggering. Through tremendous effort, I was able to maintain my high expectations for a while until burnout set in. That's when I started doubting—myself, my childhood dream, and the promise of the Lord for my life.

I had to get real with myself. It is impossible to set high standards and always expect to achieve them. This can only lead to being stressed out all the time. We are human. We will falter. We will fail. It is in our nature. However, what sets some of us apart from others is our ability to stay in the race and cross the finish line.

The following is the result of my experience coming out of burnout and assessing myself in light of my relationship with God. These are my ideals, but for each, I had to understand my place in God's grace.

Possess Deep Knowledge In My Field Of Medicine

Medical studies are overwhelming. This is because the modern age thinks that the better your knowledge of your field, the better doctor you will be. To maintain superior knowledge, however, you must stay ahead of the curve, reading new articles and papers, conducting research and learning the newest guidelines. It is constant pressure to stay at the top of your field.

Unfortunately, it is too easy to judge ourselves against impossible standards. This leads to a life of frustration and failure. I had to learn that life was never intended to be this way. Our identity is not based on our job position or level of expertise. Our identity lies in what Christ says about us, how He sees us through His unfathomable love.

The only standards upon which I evaluate my life are from God's word.

> *Before I formed you in the womb I knew you.*
>
> Jeremiah 1:5
>
> *I have called you by your name; you are Mine.*
>
> Isaiah 43:1

> *You are precious and honored in my sight... I love you.*
>
> Isaiah 43:4 NIV

Certainly, I expect the best of myself in my career. This is called *ambition*. It is healthy. Ambition is an essential motivation, but it is not my identity. The Creator of the universe knows my name and loves me. Our relationship is based on grace, not works. The reason I work hard is to please Him who deeply loves me. I do not need to gain His attention, as He has already chosen me to be His daughter.

> *For by grace you have been saved through faith, and that not of yourselves; it is the gift of God, not of works, lest anyone should boast.*
>
> Ephesians 2:8-9

God wants me to become His friend.

> *Draw near to God and He will draw near to you.*
>
> James 4:8

My strongest desire is to be called the friend of God, as were Abraham and Moses.

And the Scripture was fulfilled which says, "Abraham believed God, and it was accounted to him for righteousness." And he was called the friend of God.

James 2:23

So the Lord spoke to Moses face to face, as a man speaks to his friend.

Exodus 33:11

When I hold on to my identity in Christ, I flow with worship and praise into His merciful love. I grow closer to God and become His friend.

The Lord is a friend to those who fear him. He teaches them his covenant.

Psalm 25:14 NLT

I love how The Passion translation reveals this verse.

There's a private place reserved for the lovers of God, where they sit near him and receive the revelation-secrets of his promises.

The Message translation says:

God-friendship is for God-worshipers; they are the ones he confides in.

This is where I want to be—by the feet of Jesus, ministering to Him and loving Him like Martha's sister Mary did. I want to choose what is best. I know that this will not be taken away from me.

> *And Jesus answered and said to her, "Martha, Martha, you are worried and troubled about many things. But one thing is needed, and Mary has chosen that good part, which will not be taken away from her."*
>
> Luke 10:41

Excellent Patient-Physician Relationship

As much as my experience with the inconsiderate doctor upset me (part 1), I was impressed by the kindness and empathy of another physician. He knocked gently on each patient's door and entered wearing a smile. He introduced himself and the interns accompanying him. In cases where the patient was hurting, he erased his smile, grabbed a chair and sat next to them. Several minutes passed as he carefully explained what was going on. His words brought comfort. You could feel the atmosphere of hope breaking through.

Talking to patients is a skill. There is no single way to do it. Each patient is different, so every relationship is different. Yet the core values of a patient-physician relationship are the same—be kind and compassionate and yet professional.

I have learned how to begin a patient-doctor conversation, when to ask questions and when to listen to the patient. Some patients burst into tears and need psychological support, others become angry because they aren't satisfied with the treatment and are still sick or in pain. As a doctor, I should be wise enough to understand my patients' needs. After all, my care is patient-centered.

As much as this seems a daunting task, keep in mind that we have the honor of serving a great God, and through Him, we have the Holy Spirit living in us. By spending time with Him every day, we become more sensitive to how He wants us to act and speak. I love what the great worshiper, Kim Walker-Smith, says *"Fix your eyes on Him and listen to His voice and keep yourself in that place where just the slightest whisper is all it takes to attract your full attention and to be ready to walk with Him."*

> *My sheep hear My voice, and I know them, and they follow Me.*
>
> John 10:27

My desire in life is to live daily in the supernatural, to be so sensitive to the Holy Spirit that heaven manifests on earth, all for the glory of Jesus.

> *But we have this treasure in earthen vessels, that the excellence of the power may be of God and not of us.*
>
> 2 Corinthians 4:7

STRONG RELATIONSHIPS WITH COLLEAGUES

It is my responsibility to maintain a good relationship with my colleagues and coworkers. We are all different. That's what makes the medical community beautiful. Every person thinks differently and does things in a unique way. Therefore, I cannot impose my opinions on others. Jesus said to "love your neighbor as yourself" (Mark 12:31). When I love my neighbor unconditionally, I will be able to accept them. I love them because the Lord commanded me to do so, and because Jesus died for them as He did for me. We are all sons and daughters of the Most High God.

Our workplace becomes our second home, and we enjoy our long days together as a family. Healthy relationships are founded on doing what is best for each other before thinking of ourselves. If we are the light of the world, we cannot be hidden. Our good works must be clear to others.

> *Whoever wants to become great among you must be your servant.*
>
> Matthew 20:26 NIV

> *My little children, let us not love in word or in tongue, but in deed and in truth.*
>
> 1 John 3:18

> *Who is wise and understanding among you? Let them show it by their good life, by deeds done in the humility that comes from wisdom.*
>
> James 3:13 NIV

> *Let your light so shine before men, that they may see your good works and glorify your Father in heaven.*
>
> Matthew 5:16

ESTABLISH MY REPUTATION

At the end of the day, a doctor wants their name to be well-regarded. Medicine is a lifetime occupation, and it is the doctor's responsibility to keep their practice growing—helping patients, avoiding mistakes, growing in knowledge and teaching others. Therefore, a stellar reputation is crucial.

Often, the myriad of responsibilities can wear down a doctor. When I find that happening to me, I re-center my focus to one of thankfulness. I fix my eyes on Jesus and let Him teach me His ways because His ways are straight.

> *Trust in the Lord with all your heart,*
> *And lean not on your own understanding;*
> *In all your ways acknowledge Him,*
> *And He shall direct your paths.*

Proverbs 3:6

As I ponder upon His beauty and His promises for me, He leads me through the valleys of despair and walks with me through deep waters.

> *When you pass through the waters,*
> *I will be with you;*
> *And through the rivers*

> *they shall not overflow you.*
> *When you walk through the fire,*
> *you shall not be burned,*
> *Nor shall the flame scorch you.*

Isaiah 43:2

I want to be known as the doctor who does God's work. His work is kingdom-centered. It is righteousness, peace and joy.

> *For the kingdom of God is not eating and drinking, but righteousness and peace and joy in the Holy Spirit. For he who serves Christ in these things is acceptable to God and approved by men.*

Romans 14:17-18

What a privilege we have, as sons and daughters of God, to do what He desires through the Holy Spirit, to serve Christ and please God. I want God to be pleased with me just as He was with Jesus.

> *And the Holy Spirit descended in bodily form like a dove upon Him, and a voice came from heaven which said, "You are My beloved Son; in You I am well pleased."*

Luke 3:22

Let us live our lives to be Christ-like.

What about the approval of men? After all, peer-review is crucial in medicine. The answer is, it is a matter of priorities. I place peer approval second to God approval.

> *But seek first the kingdom of God and His righteousness, and all these things shall be added to you.*
>
> Matthew 6:33

> *Am I now trying to win the approval of human beings, or of God? Or am I trying to please people? If I were still trying to please people, I would not be a servant of Christ.*
>
> Galatians 1:10 NIV

This is the Apostle Paul, the person who also wrote Romans 14:17-18 quoted above. He makes it clear that our goal is to be servants of Christ, and that as we serve Him, we become pleasing to God and then approved by men (ref. Romans 14:18).

We weren't promised an easy life. Persecution does exist. Look at the life of Jesus. People adored Him and despised Him, eventually leading to His crucifixion while his followers wept. Yet the promises of God are sure.

> *When a man's ways please the LORD, He makes even his enemies to be at peace with him.*
>
> Proverbs 16:7
>
> *The fear of the Lord is the beginning of wisdom; a good understanding have all those who do His commandments.*
>
> Psalm 111:10

PRAYER

> *Come to Me, all you who labor and are heavy laden, and I will give you rest. Take My yoke upon you and learn from Me, for I am gentle and lowly in heart, and you will find rest for your souls. For My yoke is easy and My burden is light.*
>
> Matthew 11:28-30

Lord Jesus, as I become more and more aware of the responsibilities I have as a doctor, I come to You. I definitely cannot fulfill all the expectations of my patients, nor the ones I have set for myself. These expectations wear me down and I can't do this on my own. I place it all at the cross and I delightfully take your yoke. I want to live my life serving You. My only goal is to please You, God. Holy Spirit, I invite You in my heart. Burn in me Your desire and guide my steps so I can learn from Jesus how to be gentle and humble. I want to serve and love my patients, placing them before myself. I fully trust You and I thank You, God, for You hear my prayer and are faithful to take me deeper into Your resting place. Amen!

2
My Wilderness Journey

"Why did you allow this? Why did you put this desire in my heart?" I cried. "I know you don't want me to suffer but why did You choose me? You know I'm fragile. You knew I couldn't bear this much pressure."

Thus, became my daily prayer.

It was the worst feeling, like nothing I had experienced before. *Why did God ever give me a desire for medicine? Why didn't I like any other field of study at the university?* I lived this daily struggle for over a year. Apparently, becoming a doctor was more than studying the human body for 10-15 years and then treating diseases.

Becoming a doctor is like entering an entirely different universe. It is a calling beyond any other occupation or regular job. It is a sacrifice. It is tears and joy. It is failure or success, life or death. It is my calling.

Medicine is a fight for a healthy life for every patient. A doctor's challenge isn't just a healthy work-life balance, succeeding at work while enjoying family and friends. A doctor is a warrior in every patient's battle.

Unfortunately, none of this is taken into consideration during medical school. Medical school is great for teaching the details of the human body, but it fails to teach about life as a doctor and the physician-patient relationship. Medical school sends us to the battlefield unprepared.

Day after day, we hear of residents and doctors getting burned out, facing depression or even committing suicide. Sadly, nothing really changes. The workload remains the same, the stressors are the same, and the information we are required to learn multiplies every year.

Weight gain, restless sleep, social isolation, sadness, loss of interest in hobbies, lack of concentration, irritability—all were symptoms I used to diagnose myself with major depressive disorder. Still, reading these symptoms in a textbook could not compare to experiencing them. Those previously simple terms became my Goliath. Yes, I know. It's the story of a little boy who slew a giant with a sling, a stone and his faith in God. Yet my giant was still standing.

"God, is that Bible story even real? I believe in You and I'm standing before my giant, but I'm out of stones."

I am amazed by the story of David. He is my hero—courageous, full of faith, strong and fearless. As much as I looked up to him, I thought I was becoming fearless like him. Oh, how wrong I was! My life was falling apart. Depression was the biggest and mightiest giant I had ever faced. The very thing I studied a few months ago was now fighting me. That young medical student trained to fight depression in her patients was powerless over it herself.

I naively thought believers in Jesus couldn't fall into depression. Through Jesus, they had defeated the enemy, therefore they had defeated all his plans. Right? So, why was this happening to me?

Since age five, I wanted to help sick people. What calling is more impacting to helping them than a doctor? Jesus healed the sick. He defeated the enemy and robbed him of his power. And now Jesus was calling me to rise up and believe that the Holy Spirit still does miracles by the same divine power.

At 15 years old, the Lord confirmed my lifelong desire through a prophetic word.

"You want to become a doctor... and you will be a good doctor."

"Awesome! That is so amazing," I said to myself.

I was a believer when I received this word, a follower of Jesus and a conqueror by His powerful blood. I had authority over the enemy through Jesus' name. I was so ready to start this journey. Little did I know what awaited me—a wilderness of relentless schooling, oppressive self-doubt, internal criticism and sleepless nights pulling 24-hour shifts.

Two years prior to graduation, I started thinking about quitting. Studying wasn't "my thing" anymore. I thought to myself: *What kind of pleasure awaits me on the other side of this dream that I would choose to sacrifice 15 years of my life for?*

I was 23 years old and regretting my fate.

I didn't sign up for this. I'm a young woman ready to don her white coat and walk the hospital, a strong and confident doctor helping the suffering and infirm. That's what I signed up for. Yet here I am, barely sleeping, studying incessantly, getting poor grades, running the hallways, always behind schedule, scouring my brain for answers, filling out endless paperwork and looking like the west wind chose my wardrobe. What's that all about? I'm used to looking good. Now I've gained 10 pounds, wear scrubs all day, and have gray bags under my eyes. My high school friends are graduating from university, going out every weekend and earning money.

You got it all wrong God. This calling is not for me. You have the wrong person. I can't do this. I don't want to waste my life lost between hospital floors, seeing patients I can't cure and looking plain. Please God, remove this from my life. Please God, call me into ministry. I want to serve you. I adore you and want to dedicate my life to You. I'll do anything. Anything but this! Staying in medicine means locked in my room forever studying. I give up! Why did I ever want medicine in the first place?

For many years, I came to hear stories of doctors whom God called to leave their work and follow Him through ministry. I knew this would happen to me one day. Therefore, I thought ministry would be my only getaway.

"But why did you let these doctors study for almost 15 years before taking them to full-time ministry?" I asked God.

For that, I heard no answer.

At that moment, my life was meaningless. My lifelong dream was my worst nightmare. The very thing I longed to achieve became the thing I was trying to escape. All my life, I had set my identity in the doctor I would one day become.

Now that I lost my desire for medicine, I lost my identity and purpose in life. I lost faith in God's word that I would become a good doctor. I lost faith in myself. I became weak and lonely, sure that nobody understood what I was going through. Other medical students were happy and getting high grades. They were spending night shifts learning and there I was crying in the room during every shift.

What do I do? Is this place for me? I don't even know how to prescribe a simple painkiller. I'm not learning a thing. I'm barely surviving, fighting for every hour of sanity.

I felt so dumb! Every mistake I made in training crushed me. I couldn't stop the onslaught of self-criticism. I fell asleep crying and woke up crying. I went to work tired and returned home depressed. I prayed every day, believing I had God and that was all I needed.

The prophetic word I received as an adolescent was a strong confirmation to my childhood dream, but during these tough times, I decided that quitting was my best option. *Dedicating my life to ministry will always work out even if it is not my calling. After all, I am serving Jesus.*

I couldn't see a bad outcome to leaving medical school and getting into ministry. For me, it was a win-win situation. I would finally escape the craziness of studies, night shifts and staggering responsibilities of medicine, and I would be able to serve God in ministry.

After the diagnosis of depression, I had a new fear. According to what I learned, suicidal thoughts might accompany depression. I never had them, but I was afraid of the possibility of getting them. I love Jesus. I want to live for Him. I could not let depression be the end.

During that period of suffering, I received a second prophecy. This one was a word of encouragement to pursue what the Lord had called me to do, and to not give up on that dream. Through endless prayers and the tremendous support of my family and friends, I was able to regain some of my strength. And at the Spirit's leading, I felt to seek medical help.

God brought me to a great team. A psychiatrist and a psychotherapist worked with me until I was healthy again. Without their help, I would've never made it. As a patient, I thanked God for doctors and healthcare professionals. There I was, complaining every day about being a doctor, but now I was grateful for the medical help that changed my life.

Now I knew, from a patient's perspective, what a huge difference doctors can make! I knew the power of a physician fighting with their patient! It was tremendous!

I was ready to fight again!

A year went by, and I asked God the same question once again "Why do you allow some doctors to study and work for decades before calling them into full-time ministry?"

This time, I felt Him gently whispering "There is growth in the process."

Couldn't it be a shorter process, God? A simpler process? A smoother process?

I might not have received answers to all these questions, but I trust His perfect wisdom and understanding. I am sure the process of a medical career brings about so many changes different than what other journeys do. Compassion, caring for others, serving the families, relying on Jesus when my medical knowledge fails are few of the experiences that I don't get to learn in other careers. Yes, God might call me into a full-time ministry after years of medical practice, but I trust Him enough to know that what I went through and continue to go through are not for nothing. It is through irritation that pearls are formed, and we are some unique pearls formed through our medical journey. We have a unique color and beauty to offer the world. This type of pearls is made to show the world the unique characteristic of Jesus, the Great Physician, through us following His steps and imitating Him.

3
Completed in Christ

My recovery from depression was more than just the restoration of my mental state. I underwent a relearning of sorts, acquiring the necessary knowledge that medical school neglected. Here, in abbreviated form, is what I learned. May it help you as it did me.

1. WE ARE THE PATIENT'S HOPE.

Doctors give hope to their patients—physical, mental, emotional and spiritual hope. This is because a person is made of three parts: body, soul and spirit.

> *Now may the God of peace Himself sanctify you completely; and may your whole spirit, soul, and body be preserved blameless at the coming of our Lord Jesus Christ.*
>
> 1 Thessalonians 5:23

Body

Patients often visit a doctor as a last result. After trying their own remedies, consulting friends and family, and yes... researching on the Internet, they finally resort to seeking a trained medical professional. It's their last option, the only hope for their physical needs, and they're desperate.

Soul

Other times, patients burdened by their diseases or chronic conditions are troubled in their souls. That's where the doctor can be the patient's mental or emotional hope. In some cases, patients open up and describe personal problems with family, their jobs, or other relationship.

A common occurrence is a patient consulting for insomnia and ending up with a diagnosis of depression. Physical diseases can be rooted in emotional and mental illnesses. To treat them, I must talk to the patient and give them my full attention. This is as important as prescribing medication or performing surgery. Unfortunately, medical school does not always focus on this part of clinical assessment, but with practice and prayer, physicians eventually succeed.

Spirit

Sometimes the doctor is the patient's spiritual hope. For example, if I have a patient who doubts the existence of God but is still searching for the truth—perhaps the patient is desperate for another treatment option after medicine has failed—I might ask them: "Would you mind if I pray with you? I believe in Jesus and His healing."

Bear in mind, however, that persecution does exist. Some people could use your invitation as an opportunity to attack not just you, but Christianity as a whole.

As doctors, we have a great opportunity to offer Jesus to our patients as the best medicine. A question risks little. A prayer yields much.

> *To them God willed to make known what are the riches of the glory of this mystery among the Gentiles: which is Christ in you, the hope of glory.*
>
> Colossians 1:27

We, as sons and daughters of God, are the hope of this world because we have encountered Jesus and are filled with the Holy Spirit. The world is waiting for us to be revealed as children of God. We cannot hide anymore. The world needs hope and we are the ambassadors of Christ. We should be the ones bringing light and hope to this broken world.

> *For the earnest expectation of the creation eagerly waits for the revealing of the sons of God. For the creation was subjected to futility, not willingly, but because of Him who subjected it in hope; because the creation itself also will be delivered from the bondage of corruption into the glorious liberty of the children of God.*
>
> Romans 8:19-21

As physicians following the Great Physician, we need to see the patient as a whole person—body, soul and spirit. Rather than treating the symptoms, we must search for the cause. Sometimes, the cause of physical symptoms is psychological or spiritual. This is why we not only examine the patient's body, but also, through an understanding of a patient's history, we should examine potential emotional and/or spiritual causes.

I'm not saying that it is easy, and I'm not saying that we should push the patient to talk about everything at all times. However, by following the leading of the

Spirit, we can help the patient get a complete recovery.

I have heard of people suffering from chronic physical pain caused by bitterness or unforgiveness. As soon as they released those involved by forgiving them, the resultant spiritual freedom set them free physically as well. Spiritual healing brings physical healing.

Jesus not only healed physically broken people, but He also treated those who were mentally and spiritually oppressed.

> *God anointed Jesus of Nazareth with the Holy Spirit and with power, who went about doing good and healing all who were oppressed by the devil, for God was with Him.*
>
> Acts 10:38

Doctors work in an environment where patients are vulnerable, not only regarding their bodies but also their lives. We must be sensitive enough to detect situations where the problem is deeper than physical. We must train ourselves in how to ask the right questions at the right times.

We are great at treating physical illnesses and providing physical hope, but we ought to strive to bring hope for the soul and spirit of a patient. As children of God, we should be seeking this from the Father.

> *And whatever you ask in My name, that I will do, that the Father may be glorified in the Son.*
>
> John 14:13
>
> *May the God of hope fill you with all joy and peace as you trust in him, so that you may overflow with hope by the power of the Holy Spirit.*
>
> Romans 15:13 NIV

PRAYER

Lord, I trust in You alone. I ask You for wisdom and grace to learn how to approach my patients with the hope that You have given me. I don't want to keep Your hope for myself, but I want to overflow with it and pass it on to my patients and colleagues. Thank You for Your faithfulness. Amen!

2. Intercession

While we should not impose our beliefs on others, there are many ways to politely ask the patients if we may pray for them. If a patient refuses, we can still intercede for them in our private prayer life.

When appropriate, I ask the Holy Spirit to pray through me. However, my prayers don't end when the patients leave the room. As followers of Jesus Christ, we were called to intercede.

> *Likewise the Spirit also helps in our weaknesses. For we do not know what we should pray for as we ought, but the Spirit Himself makes intercession for us with groanings which cannot be uttered.*
>
> Romans 8:26

Having a strong relationship with the Lord cannot be hidden. All the world will see a difference in you. When you spend time with the Word and let the Holy Spirit minister to you, filling you with the fruit of the Spirit, your light will shine brightly. It will reveal to those around you that you carry God's Spirit within.

Jesus longs to be your friend. He reveals His secrets to His friends.

> *The secret of the Lord is with those who fear Him.*
>
> Psalm 25:14

Of course, we don't spend time with Jesus to get secrets. We spend time with Jesus because He is the Holy One, the King of Kings, the Lord of Lords, the Risen One, our deliverer, savior, the love of our lives, the living God who bankrupted heaven to come and save us because that's how much He is in love with each of us.

Remarkably, when a friend of God enters His presence, the communication is two-way. The friend speaks and God listens. Likewise, God speaks and the friend listens. Each has a right to give and take. Consider Abraham who was called the friend of God.

> *Then the men turned away from there and went toward Sodom, but Abraham still stood before the Lord. And Abraham came near and said, "Would You also destroy the righteous with the wicked?... So the Lord said... Then Abraham answered... So the Lord went His way as soon as He finished speaking with Abraham; and Abraham returned to his place.*
>
> Genesis 18:22-33

Abraham spoke up six times regarding Sodom, and the Lord replied six times. The effect of the exchange was profound.

> *And it came to pass, when God destroyed the cities of the plain, that God remembered Abraham, and sent Lot out of the midst of the overthrow, when He overthrew the cities in which Lot had dwelt.*
>
> Genesis 19:29

This is intercession. Abraham was praying, talking to God on behalf of the few righteous people in Sodom. And the Lord heard His friend's prayer and acted accordingly.

What a powerful calling it is to intercede! And from whom do we get our reward? From God alone.

> *And whatever you do, do it heartily, as to the Lord and not to men, knowing that from the Lord you will receive the reward of the inheritance; for you serve the Lord Christ.*
>
> Colossians 3:23-24

> *Therefore, my beloved brethren, be steadfast, immovable, always abounding in the work of*

> *the Lord, knowing that your labor is not in vain in the Lord.*
>
> 1 Corinthians 15:58

In chapter 1, we talked about our responsibility as doctors to care for a patient's health. But our responsibility goes beyond this. As Christian doctors, we should intercede for our patients the way we intercede for our families and friends. In my practice, I ask the Lord to give me words of knowledge to my patients. I ask Him for wisdom to speak to their hearts and for boldness in sharing the gospel of Jesus with them. I have a great opportunity to reclaim their souls back to the Lord. I want to take time and pray for their healing, that the Lord alone will be glorified through it.

In interceding, we lift the patient's mental, emotional and physical needs. However, it is crucial to leave those burdens at the cross of Jesus. It is not our responsibility to carry them. The price was paid once and for all, for them and for us. We are just the patients' helpers. We need Jesus as much as they do.

> *Casting all your care upon Him, for He cares for you.*
>
> 1 Peter 5:7

I take time at the end of my shift to pray for the patients that I saw that day. In the morning, I often pray for the patients who will be visiting me. My prayer could be as simple and genuine as "Lord, help them find You, speak to their hearts, use me to show them who You really are."

I also fast for a few days every month, praying for all the patients I saw or will be seeing during that time. The Lord knows them one by one. Fasting opens heaven for us to receive the breakthrough of a healing ministry.

> *And He said to them, "Go into all the world and preach the gospel to every creature. He who believes and is baptized will be saved; but he who does not believe will be condemned. And these signs will follow those who believe: In My name they will cast out demons; they will speak with new tongues; they will take up serpents; and if they drink anything deadly, it will by no means hurt them; they will lay hands on the sick, and they will recover."*
>
> Mark 16:15-18

Jesus was not *suggesting* that we go into all the world. This was a command to "Go!" And because we love Jesus, we obey His commands. Not only that, but if we obey His commands, we will remain in His love.

> *Jesus answered and said to him, "If anyone loves Me, he will keep My word; and My Father will love him, and We will come to him and make Our home with him. He who does not love Me does not keep My words; and the word which you hear is not Mine but the Father's who sent Me.*
>
> John 14:23-24

> *If you keep My commandments, you will abide in My love, just as I have kept My Father's commandments and abide in His love.*
>
> John 15:10

After His command, Jesus gave us a promise.

> *They will lay hands on the sick, and they will recover.*
>
> Mark 16:18

Jesus also gave another command.

> *Heal the sick, cleanse the lepers, raise the dead, cast out demons. Freely you have received, freely give.*
>
> Matthew 10:8

This again was not a suggestion. God's promise never fails, so the sick will get healed when I pray for them. It is the Father's will that they recover.

Preaching the gospel and healing the sick were the works of Jesus on earth. We are to follow His lead.

> *Then Jesus went about all the cities and villages, teaching in their synagogues, preaching the gospel of the kingdom, and healing every sickness and every disease among the people.*
>
> Matthew 9:35

So, what happens when our prayers seemingly don't work? I believe that in the cases where the patients don't get healed, the problem may not lie with the patient's faith, as we may believe. The problem could be with our faith. In Mark, it is written that "these signs (one of which is healing) will accompany those who believe." *Those who believe* means us.

Remember the father in Matthew 17 who brought his son who had seizures to the disciples. He had faith that they would heal the boy in the name of Jesus, but Jesus ended up blaming the disciples when the boy was not delivered. He did not blame the father nor the child. Instead, He charged His most ardent followers, the future of His kingdom message, with a lack of faith:

> *So Jesus said to them, "Because of your unbelief; for assuredly, I say to you, if you have faith as a mustard seed, you will say to this mountain, 'Move from here to there,' and it will move; and nothing will be impossible for you.*
>
> Matthew 17:20

Not only should we hang on to a bold faith, but we should also pray and fast with consistency.

> *Then Jesus told his disciples a parable to show them that they should always pray and not give up.*
>
> Luke 18:1 NIV

> *However, this kind does not go out except by prayer and fasting.*
>
> Matthew 17:21

We should strive to get more of Jesus and let the Holy Spirit fill us each day. Only then will we be ready to pour into others.

3. Learn From Jesus

My one true desire is to be like Jesus, the Great Physician, and to follow His lead, not only in medicine but in every aspect of life. Nothing else matters in this world than to make Him proud.

Few years ago, while praying, I had a vision of myself as a little girl shadowing her father who was a doctor working in the Intensive Care Unit of a hospital. The father was Jesus. Since then, I constantly pray and ask Jesus that from the day I start residency until the day I retire, to never leave my side. I want to be the student of the Great Physician, to give Him all my weaknesses and retrieve from Him wisdom and knowledge. Only after my surrender and God's outpouring, will I be able to care for my patients.

In life, never be content with what you know. Never stop learning because life is never done teaching.

This is exactly what I want to be doing. I want to learn to become more like Jesus—how He prayed, how He healed the sick, how He raised the dead, how He loved those who persecuted Him, how He resisted the devil, how He served others putting them first so He could be the best leader, how He endured hardship fixing His eyes on the joy that's ahead, etc.

> *Therefore we also, since we are surrounded by so great a cloud of witnesses, let us lay aside every weight, and the sin which so easily ensnares us, and let us run with endurance the race that is set before us, looking unto Jesus, the author and finisher of our faith, who for the joy that was set before Him endured the cross, despising the shame, and has sat down at the right hand of the throne of God. For consider Him who endured such hostility from sinners against Himself, lest you become weary and discouraged in your souls.*
>
> Hebrews 12:1-3

JESUS' PRAYER LIFE

A key component of Jesus' life on earth was prayer. Without His connection with the Father, the man Jesus could never have fulfilled His divine purpose here on earth, which was to save us all and redeem us to the

Father. He would not have done all the signs and wonders He did if it wasn't for His prayer time.

Consider just a small portion of the scriptural evidence.

> *So He Himself often withdrew into the wilderness and prayed.*
>
> Luke 5:16

> *And when He had sent the multitudes away, He went up on the mountain by Himself to pray. Now when evening came, He was alone there.*
>
> Matthew 14:23

> *Now it came to pass in those days that He went out to the mountain to pray, and continued all night in prayer to God.*
>
> Luke 6:12

> *Now in the morning, having risen a long while before daylight, He went out and departed to a solitary place; and there He prayed.*
>
> Mark 1:35

> *And it happened, as He was alone praying...*
>
> Luke 9:18

And He said to His disciples, "Sit here while I pray."

Mark 14:32

Now it came to pass, as He was praying in a certain place, ...

Luke 11:1

But I have prayed for you, that your faith should not fail; ...

Luke 22:32

But He, because He continues forever, has an unchangeable priesthood. Therefore He is also able to save to the uttermost those who come to God through Him, since He always lives to make intercession for them.

Hebrews 7:24-25

Who is he who condemns? It is Christ who died, and furthermore is also risen, who is even at the right hand of God, who also makes intercession for us.

Romans 8:34

And I will pray the Father, and He will give you another Helper, that He may abide with you forever.

John 14:16

Pray and declare God's truths. Proclaim Bible verses and claim God's promises over your life. Repeat over and over again the prophetic words you have received. Speak life over yourself and your family. There is power in God's Word, and there is power in your spoken word.

> *So shall My word be that goes forth from My mouth; it shall not return to Me void, but it shall accomplish what I please, and it shall prosper in the thing for which I sent it.*
>
> Isaiah 55:11

When we pray and ask the Father for something, He responds in four different ways:

Yes, and it will happen now.

Yes, but it will not happen now.

Yes, but it will not happen according to your way.

No, it won't happen.

Bold faith is expressed in different ways. Sometimes, bold faith is thanking God for answering a prayer before He answers.

> *This is the reason I urge you to boldly believe for whatever you ask for in prayer – be convinced that you have received it and it will be yours.*
>
> Mark 11:24 TPT

Other times, bold faith is a completely surrendered heart that is willing to endure the troubles of life because you trust God's sovereignty. Remember Jesus' prayer at Gethsemane. He said "Nevertheless, not as I will, but as You will" (Matthew 26:39). I know and trust that He is omniscient, omnipotent and omnipresent. He is Abba (Father), El Shaddai (God Almighty), El Olam (the Everlasting God), Yahweh Yireh (the Lord will provide), Yahweh Rophe (the Lord who heals).

God delights in a grateful heart. He loves to hear your thanksgiving. Even if you have requests, never let those surpass your thanksgiving. As King David used to tell his soul to bless the Lord, so you can also teach your soul to thank God always and in all times.

> *My soul, wait silently for God alone,*
> *For my expectation is from Him.*
>
> Psalm 62:5

Be anxious for nothing, but in everything by prayer and supplication, with thanksgiving, let your requests be made known to God.

Philippians 4:6

As you therefore have received Christ Jesus the Lord, so walk in Him, rooted and built up in Him and established in the faith, as you have been taught, abounding in it with thanksgiving.

Colossians 2:6-7

Continue earnestly in prayer, being vigilant in it with thanksgiving.

Colossians 4:2

JESUS' CARE FOR OTHERS

Many questions come to my mind when I think of Jesus' life on earth. How did He pray? How much time did He spend in prayer? How did He intercede for people? What did He usually do before, while and after He healed the sick (body, soul and spirit)? What did He tell His disciples to do when praying and interceding for the sick?

> *Therefore be imitators of God as dear children. And walk in love, as Christ also has loved us and given Himself for us, an offering and a sacrifice to God for a sweet-smelling aroma.*
>
> Ephesians 5:1-2

Jesus sometimes healed in unusual, even inappropriate ways compared to the social norms of the day. He spit in the dust, made mud and put it on the eyes of a blind man (ref. John 9:6). He left Lazarus in the grave for four days before coming and reviving him. *Why, Jesus? What's the point? You could've just said a word, up close or from afar and the people would have been healed.* Yet His position is clear.

> *I love the Father and do exactly what my Father has commanded me.*
>
> John 14:31 NIV

The 'why' is not always ours to know. The Lord is looking for obedient hearts. He is longing for generations of "Davids." The Father's desire is to have all the believers called "women and men after God's own heart."

> *Has the Lord as great delight in burnt offerings and sacrifices, as in obeying the*

> *voice of the Lord? Behold, to obey is better than sacrifice, and to heed than the fat of rams.*
>
> 1 Samuel 15:22

> *Obey My voice, and I will be your God, and you shall be My people. And walk in all the ways that I have commanded you, that it may be well with you.*
>
> Jeremiah 7:23

Jesus the man was obedient to God the Father unto death. His prayer for our salvation prevailed over His prayer to escape death. It was because He prayed 'not my will but yours' that God heard Him. His submission to the Father and His godly fear led Him to be raised and glorified.

> *Who, in the days of His flesh, when He had offered up prayers and supplications, with vehement cries and tears to Him who was able to save Him from death, and was heard because of His godly fear, though He was a Son, yet He learned obedience by the things which He suffered. And having been perfected, He became the author of eternal salvation to all who obey Him*
>
> Hebrews 5:7-9

Jesus left His heavenly throne and came to earth to love and save us. On the day of the last supper, He washed His disciples' feet to teach them humility.

How much more must we follow His example daily with the people who surround us? Our lives should speak on Jesus' behalf because the Holy Spirit lives in us. We are not who the world says we are. We are sons and daughters of the Most High. I don't want to be recognized as the best doctor who has great knowledge but has a bad attitude, who doesn't know how to talk to people, who isn't attentive to them or discriminates between the patients.

I want to be remembered as the doctor through whom we saw Jesus Christ, the doctor who served with all her heart and followed Jesus' example. I want to learn from Jesus, to pray for people and give them the best that I have. I have the King of Kings and Lord of Lords as my savior and my best friend. That is what I want to show the world.

I want to learn Jesus' steps to healing people. I want a deeper relationship with God, hearing His voice whenever He speaks. His voice is so gentle that not everybody hears it. I want to be sensitive to His words and work accordingly.

4- What Bothers You Matters

Look at what Jesus did when a man with leprosy fell to the ground and begged him for healing:

> *Jesus reached out his hand and touched the man. "I am willing," he said. "Be clean!" And immediately the leprosy left him.*
>
> Luke 5:13

The Bible says of those who follow Jesus:

> *They will be supernaturally protected from snakes and from drinking anything poisonous. And they will lay hands on the sick and heal them.*
>
> Mark 16:18 TPT

As Christian doctors, we should be willing to do the things other doctors won't do. Nobody would touch a man with leprosy. I can imagine if this man came to Jesus' disciples to get healing, they would have probably not touched him, but instead prayed for him from a distance. How about we take a step forward, follow Jesus and do the impossible in the eyes of man?

I am not just referring to touching the leprous. What I am saying is, because of our identity in Christ and the authority He has imparted in us, we have the divine power supporting and protecting us. Even if the step we take will lead us to persecution, let the Word of God win over our circumstances.

On one of my first night shifts as a medical student, the Lord put on my heart to pray for a specific patient. It was past midnight and I had just climbed into bed when I started thinking about that patient. He was severely disabled and had spent most of his life in and out of hospitals. He was always accompanied by his mother who took constant care of him. I didn't know them; I had just seen them that night for a few minutes after he was hospitalized.

As I was trying to sleep, I felt the Holy Spirit tell me to go back to his room and pray for him. I was exhausted!

"Please God, not now. I want to sleep a bit before they call me again," I said. Still, the urge got stronger and stronger, and every time I pleaded: "Not now God, what am I going to tell them? Why me? I never prayed for the sick. What am I supposed to say?"

After 40 minutes of me pleading my case, God's Word prevailed over my excuses. Thank God! I couldn't find sleep, which ironically was the main point of me rejecting the word in the first place. I went to the patient's room and asked his mother—who was sitting up with him—if I could pray for her son. I could feel her eyes scream: "Please do!"

I said a simple prayer for the Lord to heal him and protect him and his family. Then I thanked the mom and ran back to my room. Being new to this (and being a bit of a perfectionist), I was stressed that I might have messed up the ministry opportunity, said the wrong words or did some other mistake. Yet my joy was beyond explanation.

The patient didn't get well physically, at least not instantaneously. I did not follow up on him, but I could not forget the power and joy I experienced in that moment. I was finally able to partner with the Holy Spirit and obey His voice instead of letting my words prevail. It took a lot of courage to do so, and the Lord honors His servant's obedience.

In life, everything needs practice. Tuning your heart to what the Holy Spirit is telling you and praying for the sick requires practice, and a lot of it. The patient in my example was not responsive, as he had an intellectual disability as well, so my prayer was succinct. But the scenario between God and me happened a couple of times again, both with conscious and responsive patients who were severely sick. They both died in the next few days after I prayed for them, but during my prayers, I had the opportunity to lead them to Christ.

It wasn't easy. I fought with the Holy Spirit in both cases, explaining passionately to God why I shouldn't be praying for these people. But thank God for His new mercies every day. Thank God for the fire He puts inside of us that could not be tamed, because if it was, those patients could've died without hearing my proclamation of the truth that Jesus is Lord. I might have been the first to pray for them... or maybe the last. They clearly did not recover physically but I can never know what God stirred in their spirits that moment. It is God's responsibility to check their hearts. As for me, God is looking for obedience. He delights when His child says, "on account of Your Word, God, I will obey because You are the good and faithful Father."

Those few times, it was the Holy Spirit who nudged my heart to pray for the sick.

FAILURE

I remember another time when my friend asked me to accompany her to pray for another friend. She was dying from cancer. Now, I had the time to prepare myself. I was able to pray for the friend before actually praying with her. Unlike the previous experiences when I responded to impromptu directions from the Holy Spirit, I felt ready in this case.

We visited the friend twice that week. We prayed for her salvation and her healing, but she died after a few days. It was heartbreaking. During that period, I was on fire for Jesus and constantly asking Him to put patients in my path to pray for them. Having my friend ask me to pray for that person was so unexpected, it felt like a divine appointment to experience a miracle. Yet after intercession and fervent prayers, she died.

I knew this could never be a reason to stop praying for the sick. On the contrary, this was an invitation to go back to my secret place in God's presence and pray even more for His resurrection power to manifest through me, all for His glory.

Never underestimate the power of your prayers and the drastic changes that are often invisible. I am extremely blessed to be able to ask the Lord to mold me more like Him.

When you read about the great women and men of God who saw hundreds and thousands of healing miracles, their stories always began with "failures." But what we perceive as a failure is growth in God's eyes. It represents one step closer to the breakthrough. By obeying His words, we are empowering our faith and our spiritual authority... one prayer at a time.

Heidi Baker, Bill Johnson and Randy Clark are few modern-day heroes through whom God performed mighty healing miracles. Yet don't be intimidated by their testimonies. They started the same place we are starting. And because of their obedience and complete surrender to Christ, they were able to experience mighty healing revivals.

Look up to these people and learn from their mistakes. And when it comes to loving your patients, love them perfectly. Love is the key for every breakthrough, especially in the healing ministry.

> *Since you are children of a perfect Father in heaven, you are to be perfect like him.*
>
> Matthew 5:48 TPT

FAITH

As I learned to walk as others have walked, I had to confront my own apparent weakness of faith. I asked God: "Lord, I know that You are the healer and that the same power that did miracles in the Bible is living in me now. How can I keep praying for the sick when three out of four patients I prayed for died?"

His response was clear.

> *Now faith is the substance of things hoped for, the evidence of things not seen.*
>
> Hebrews 11:1

In my question, there was a thing hoped for—to pray for the sick. There was also the substance to it—my declaration that Jesus is the Healer and His power lives in me. This is faith.

As long as the things I hope for are consistent with the Word of God, proclaiming them, putting words or substance to that hope, that is a declaration of faith.

"The evidence of things not seen" is seen. So, faith is seen by my reactions to the circumstances, by the words I speak and by the thoughts I think.

> *But without faith it is impossible to please Him, for he who comes to God must believe that He is, and that He is a rewarder of those who diligently seek Him.*
>
> Hebrews 11:6

I realized that it is not enough to have a thought if I don't work it out loud. If I have an amazing invention that can change the world but don't make it reality, it is vain. Unless I put substance to the creative thought, the world won't be affected, and it will be a useless idea. In the same way, my hope is useless until I turn it into substance, into something credible, palpable and visible, whether spiritually or materially.

> *By faith Noah, being divinely warned of things not yet seen, moved with godly fear, prepared an ark for the saving of his household...*
>
> Hebrews 11:7

Noah had never seen an ark, a boat or any other waterborne vessel. Indeed, he had never seen rain. But God gave him a revelation, and by faith he made the unseen seen. This saved him and his family and ultimately, all of mankind.

We need godly boldness in our daily lives. As children of God, we want the supernatural to invade the natural. We pray "Your kingdom come, Your will be done, on earth as it is in heaven." But if we don't aim towards this proclamation, our prayer is vain. We are the workers and the harvest is ready. We are the ones who should take the Kingdom everywhere we go. The Kingdom is at hand (ref. Matthew 4:17). Let us not be ashamed of the name of Jesus. Indeed, if I want to boast about something, let it be about the cross.

> *But God forbid that I should boast except in the cross of our Lord Jesus Christ, by whom the world has been crucified to me, and I to the world.*
>
> Galatians 6:14

What Matters

One morning, I woke up repeating this sentence "What bothers you matters, what bothers you matters!" I asked the Lord what He meant by that, and I felt He was pointing out to me two chapters of this book that I had already written. They were about my responsibilities as a doctor and praying for the sick.

Sometimes we feel we are not strong enough to carry such responsibilities, that we don't know if it is the right time to pray for the sick or if they will get healed.

However, know that doubt is not from God. So whenever these doubts come to your mind, they are an attack from the enemy. He is trying his best to stop you from doing the Lord's will and from reaching the top. Always remember your identity in Christ.

"If you teach people to heal the sick, raise the dead and cast out demons and you don't teach them who they are, then they have a performance-based identity. But as soon as you figure out who you are, you're like 'if that's who I am, where's my power?'... You are a child of God." ~ Kris Vallotton

When Jesus prayed for the believers, He said "And the glory which You gave Me I have given them, that they may be one just as We are one" (John 17:22).

I am the righteousness of God. I have the Holy Spirit living inside of me.

> *Most assuredly, I say to you, he who believes in Me, the works that I do he will do also; and greater works than these he will do, because I go to My Father. And whatever you ask in My name, that I will do, that the Father may be glorified in the Son. If you ask anything in My name, I will do it.*
>
> John 14:12-14

We have been given the authority to move mountains and change the world around us. We just need a "mustard seed" size of faith to do so. We have the Resurrection power living inside of us. We have the Holy Spirit, "The Helper" who is from God the Father.

> *But the Helper, the Holy Spirit, whom the Father will send in My name, He will teach you all things, and bring to your remembrance all things that I said to you.*
>
> John 14:26

The Holy Spirit is the full Presence of God, both on earth and within every believer. He is the comforter, the promised Holy Spirit, the breath of God, the spirit of Truth.

> *But when the Helper comes, whom I shall send to you from the Father, the Spirit of truth who proceeds from the Father, He will testify of Me.*
>
> John 15:26

> *In Him you also trusted, after you heard the word of truth, the gospel of your salvation; in whom also, having believed, you were sealed with the Holy Spirit of promise,*
>
> Ephesians 1:13

> *However, when He, the Spirit of truth, has come, He will guide you into all truth; for He will not speak on His own authority, but whatever He hears He will speak; and He will tell you things to come.*
>
> John 16:13

As a bride is precious to her bridegroom, so are we in the eyes of the Lord. The Bible says that the man who finds a wife finds a treasure (ref. Proverbs 18:22). My identity lies in who Christ says I am. He calls me chosen, forgiven, redeemed and loved by the Most High God. So, as His beloved child, I can do what He says I can do, and I inherit His Power that now flows through me.

> *Follow God's example, therefore, as dearly loved children and walk in the way of love, just as Christ loved us and gave himself up for us as a fragrant offering and sacrifice to God.*
>
> Ephesians 5:1-2

PRAYER

All I want to do is follow You Jesus! You are so worthy of all my attention and all my love. You are so worthy to take all the glory and all the honor. Yours is all dominion and power. Thank you for your never-ending, everlasting, unconditional and relentless love.

Lord, Your specialty is the miraculous. You are the One and only physician who is an expert in this field, and today I choose this same field. I want to follow You and learn from You.

> *For I am not ashamed of the gospel, because it is the power of God that brings salvation to everyone who believes...*
>
> Romans 1:16

4
Trusting God

Like most driven people, I have a tendency to see the lack in myself while observing the extraordinary ability of others. This even happened when I was first in my class in school.

This has led to some interesting conversations with my Creator.

How is it possible that you chose me, God?

Why do you want to use this broken vessel?

I am not enough. I was never enough.

Yeah, never a good idea to compare yourself to others. Marianne Williamson puts it best.

"Our deepest fear is not that we are inadequate. Our deepest fear is that we are powerful beyond measure. It is our light, not our darkness that most frightens us. We ask ourselves, 'Who am I to be brilliant, gorgeous, talented, fabulous?' Actually, who are you not to be?

You are a child of God. Your playing small does not serve the world. There is nothing enlightened about shrinking so that other people won't feel insecure around you. We are all meant to shine, as children do. We were born to make manifest the glory of God that is within us. It's not just in some of us; it's in everyone. And as we let our own light shine, we unconsciously give other people permission to do the same. As we are liberated from our own fear, our presence automatically liberates others."

I first read this passage back in 2013, and since then have read it over and over again until it became part of me. When God puts a big dream in your heart and you know it is true, yet you are afraid to admit it, proclaim this quote until you embrace its truth.

My playing small does not serve the world. I am a child of God.

Pastor Bill Johnson says (paraphrasing) "Jesus was the humblest man who ever walked the face of the earth. How many times did He criticize Himself? Never."

I was created in the image of God, made to be as humble as He is. Being humble has nothing to do with belittling myself. Even a king in all his glory can be humble while still defeating the enemy and ruling over many nations.

Consider Jesus, the King of kings. He is the lamb who was slain before the foundation of the world, yet He reigns over all the universe in glory and majesty. And as a child of God, we have His favor and the favor of others. As we learn to live out the liberty He has given us, we will help others get free as well.

I never thought I would be writing a book. What do I have to share? I am in no way an expert in any field. In fact, when God put a desire in my heart to write, I was in my lowest pit, fighting depression and everything that was coming against His promises for my life. So, I asked Him what He wanted it to be about.

He said, "What does it mean to fully trust God?"

That answer was the beginning of my healing from depression. Those few words sparked a fire in my soul to begin writing. I searched the Bible for passages about trusting God. How did the heroes of faith trust God? In the next couple of years, I absorbed hundreds of messages on trusting God. It was my "five loaves and two fishes" moment. I gave them to Jesus to bless and multiply.

"Here it is God," I whispered. "My life is a complete mess, but I have Your promise and I give it back to You to bless and multiply."

My trust journey increased daily. One day, I trusted Him for strength to go to work in the midst of my depression. Another day, I trusted Him to guide my steps to leave my home country, Lebanon, and move to the U.S. These were victorious moments, but there were many setbacks in between. However, when I made mistakes in my limited capacities, I trusted Him all the more for His mercies and grace to take my ashes and turn them into beauty. This is who my God is. He is the God of abundance! He promised that I would live in the overflow, the more than enough, because He is my all-sufficiency.

As I look back at my beautiful experiences, my "I am not enough" turned into "You are more than enough for me because Your grace is sufficient. When I am weak, You are my strength."

Hallelujah!

Here are some things I learned as part of God's restoration of my self-image. It's hard to feel bad about yourself when you understand that you are worth the price of His son.

1. Fill Your Cup

Every Christian should expect to hear these words from their Savior at the end of their life.

> *Well done, good and faithful servant; you have been faithful over a few things, I will make you ruler over many things.*
>
> Matthew 25:23

God not only wants doctors to take care of their patients; He also wants doctors to take care of themselves.

Prior to becoming medical doctors, we only had to care for ourselves. Then, throughout residency and fellowship, we are entrusted with more than ourselves. Yet how we treat those lives and our own determines how much we will be entrusted in the future.

Don't take your life for granted. Eat healthily, sleep well, enjoy a few weeks of vacation, spend time with your family and friends. But most importantly, spend time with the Lord—in His Word, worshiping Him, praying and having fellowship with other believers. This is the expression of our Christian life. There's nothing better than living this way.

Your life is extremely precious to Jesus. He bought it with His own blood. He called you righteous instead of sinner, clothed you with goodness for your iniquities, and gave you peace and good health.

> *But He was wounded for our transgressions,*
> *He was bruised for our iniquities;*
> *The chastisement for our peace was upon Him,*
> *And by His stripes we are healed.*
>
> Isaiah 53:5

> *Or do you not know that your body is the temple of the Holy Spirit who is in you, whom you have from God, and you are not your own? For you were bought at a price; therefore glorify God in your body and in your spirit, which are God's.*
>
> 1 Corinthians 6:19-20

As a Christian, when I accept Jesus as my Lord and Savior, my body becomes the temple of the Holy Spirit. Therefore, I should take care of my body and treat it as a carrier of God's Holy presence. When the Lord sees how well I am taking care of my life, He will promote me and "put me in charge of many things," which in this context is being responsible for patients' lives.

Being healthy isn't merely related to the body. Health has many components: physical, mental, psychological and spiritual. In the first chapter, we talked about the three parts of a person: body, soul and spirit. Each of these requires health. I am not saying this is easy, in fact it is a big challenge to achieve good health in all three areas of a human life. However, the Holy Spirit is our Helper. When we surrender everything to Him, He will make all things new, guiding us into the fullness of our being.

> *Keep trusting in the Lord and do what is right in his eyes. Fix your heart on the promises of God and you will be secure, feasting on his faithfulness.*
>
> Psalm 37:3 TPT

Medicine is hard. Studies are never-ending. Work is a huge responsibility. But if I am not reconciled with myself, I won't be able to study my best, work my best, and most importantly serve and love others as myself. I cannot pour from an empty cup. If I want to fulfill my calling and give the best I have, my cup should be full.

How is that possible?

When I understand how much God loves me and is taking care of me, I cannot help but love myself, believe in myself and be confident in who He is calling me to be.

> *The Lord is my shepherd; I shall not want. He makes me to lie down in green pastures; He leads me beside the still waters. He restores my soul; He leads me in the paths of righteousness for his name's sake. Yea, though I walk through the valley of the shadow of death, I will fear no evil; for You are with me; Your rod and Your staff, they comfort me. You prepare a table before me in the presence of my enemies; You anoint my head with oil; my cup runs over. Surely goodness and mercy shall follow me all the days of my life; and I will dwell in the house of the Lord forever.*

Psalm 23:1-6

Jesus is my everything. As I fix my eyes on Him, I find all I need in His Perfect nature. He is the bread of life that satisfies me. He is the living water that brings peace and restoration. He is my refuge and my strength. He is the way, the truth, and the life.

For of Him and through Him and to Him are all things.

Romans 11:36

In order to pour into others, I must first fill my cup by declaring Jesus King, reading the Word of God, dwelling in the Presence of the Lord, being filled with the Holy Spirit, and trusting God at all times.

As each one has received a gift, minister it to one another, as good stewards of the manifold grace of God.

1 Peter 4:10

2. STUDY AND WORK WILL NEVER END

"There's not one part of our lives that is worthy of hopelessness." ~ Bill Johnson

Once you choose medicine, you will never be done with studies and work. And yet life is so much more than this. We were created for greater things. We were handmade by the Creator of the universe to worship Him, adore Him, and tell the whole world that Jesus is King. He redeemed our lives so we could live eternally with Him. The few decades we have on earth are nothing compared to the eternity we are promised in the presence of the King of kings.

To endure this busy lifestyle of medicine while keeping our focus on God, we need to trust the Prince of Peace.

> *You will keep him in perfect peace, whose mind is stayed on You, because he trusts in You.*
>
> Isaiah 26:3

Each person has a calling that the Lord established for them long before their birth. It is up to you to choose this calling and to walk with Christ every single moment. The alternative is to choose anything else you want and not have your full potential and divine blessings over you. But remember, on the last day, you will be judged and give an account according to what you were called to do, not according to what you did.

> *Therefore, brethren, be even more diligent to make your call and election, for if you do these things you will never stumble; for so an entrance will be supplied to you abundantly into the everlasting kingdom of our Lord and Savior Jesus Christ.*
>
> 2 Peter 1:10-11

For the gifts and the calling of God are irrevocable.

Romans 11:29

For we are His workmanship, created in Christ Jesus to do good works, which God prepared beforehand that we should walk in them.

Ephesians 2:10

Who knows when their time on earth is due? Nobody can predict whether they are going to live 20 more years or 20 more minutes. With that in mind, have you settled your account with God? Have you asked Jesus to be your Lord and Savior? He alone can move your spirit's destiny from eternal death to eternal life in a blink of an eye. All He desires is for you to know Him as the almighty and loving God that He is. Our Father is so compassionate towards us, His children. We are His masterpieces. He loved us unto the death of Jesus on the cross to save us and restore us to Him.

I won't carry anything with me to eternity except the souls I was given to pour into and the obedience I lived in. No matter how hard I work, there will be people wiser, richer, happier and more satisfied. And no matter how hard I work, there will be much more to be done, more books to be written, more subjects to be studied, more mountains to be climbed.

> *Of making many books there is no end, and much study is wearisome to the flesh.*
>
> Ecclesiastes 12:12

Studies and work will never satisfy my hunger and thirst for God. But we have Jesus, the living water and the bread of life, who satisfies our souls.

The road to eternal life is so narrow. And our time on earth is fleeting. Let us not waste our time on meaningless things but be wise with the time we are given. I am not saying we should not work or study. On the contrary, doctors are called to do so. What I am saying is, we should fulfill God's calling on our lives at all times by taking His Kingdom wherever we go and glorifying His name in everything we do.

Let us not wait for church services or prayer meetings to serve God. The hospitals and clinics are our pulpits. We have this amazing privilege to serve patients and coworkers and show them the love of Christ.

3. Bitter To Sweet

Throughout the period of depression, questioning God's calling for my life and wrestling with my thoughts left me broken. The most bitter thing was ignoring the prophetic word I had received nine years prior. If it wasn't for that word, I would have easily quit, and I could supposedly find happiness in my life again. But that prophetic word was burning on the inside. I knew I shouldn't disobey God, but medicine was a nightmare.

In my defeated state, I thought that by staying in medical school, I would never have a ministry where I could share Jesus with the world. However, the Lord corrected me and is still correcting me every day, showing me that He is over everything and how, by seeking first His kingdom in my life, nothing will be impossible.

Let me put it this way: when I focus on anything but the kingdom, the pieces of my life scatter. But as soon as I recalibrate and focus on Jesus, it is as if all the puzzle pieces are magnetically attracted together and they all fall into place. Suddenly, my life turns from "nothing is right" to "everything is perfectly imperfect" because Jesus reigns in my life.

> *He is before all things, and in him all things hold together.*
>
> Colossians 1:17 NIV

Looking back on those tough moments and seeing how far the Lord brought me, I realize that He turned every bitterness into sweetness. The prophecy that burnt my heart was the very treatment for my depression. The enemy has only one goal, which is to keep me away from God's perfect plans for my life. By holding on to God's promises, I was able to defeat Satan and regain the vision of my amazing calling. I am so precious to Jesus. I matter. Who I am matters and what I do matters.

Jesus' calling for your life may not be sweet in the beginning. You will be tested and proven. God wants to see that He is all you seek, that He is all you need in this life. And when you give your all just to be with Him, the sweetness and greatness of His calling will find you.

During that unpleasant year, I used to beg God daily to take His calling from my life and give it to someone else. I used to cry and ask God to remove my love for medicine from my heart. Thank God He never did! Now I realize that the moment you start begging God to remove His calling from your life, that is when you are the closest to your breakthrough!

> *For our light affliction, which is but for a moment, is working for us a far more exceeding and eternal weight of glory, while we do not look at the things which are seen, but at the things which are not seen. For the things which are seen are temporary, but the things which are not seen are eternal.*
>
> 2 Corinthians 4:17-18

Let us stop being impressed by the size of our problems and instead become aware of who our God is and our identity in Him.

> *But those who wait on the Lord shall renew their strength; they shall mount up with wings like eagles, they shall run and not be weary, they shall walk and not faint.*
>
> Isaiah 40:31

When you feel that you've given your all and that you've sacrificed more than you ever thought you could, remember Abraham. In obedience to God, he was about to sacrifice his only beloved son. Isaac was God's promise, born from a miracle when Abraham was 100 years old and Sarah was 90 years old.

Previously, the Lord had promised Abraham that through Isaac, Abraham's offspring would be as numerous as the stars in the sky.

> *Then He brought him outside and said, "Look now toward heaven, and count the stars if you are able to number them." And He said to him, "So shall your descendants be."*
>
> Genesis 15:5

> *But God said to Abraham, ... "Whatever Sarah has said to you, listen to her voice; for in Isaac your seed shall be called."*
>
> Genesis 21:12

So how did Abraham reckon that promise with the command to kill his son? Abraham believed that the Lord is faithful and that He would get Isaac back from the dead.

Notice the "we" in verse 5.

> *And Abraham said to his young men, "Stay here with the donkey; the lad and I will go yonder and worship, and we will come back to you."*
>
> Genesis 22:5

> *By faith Abraham, when he was tested, offered up Isaac, and he who had received the promises offered up his only begotten son, of whom it was said, "In Isaac your seed shall be called," concluding that God was able to raise him up, even from the dead, from which he also received him in a figurative sense.*
>
> Hebrews 11:17-19

You might be feeling that you have given your life up for medicine, that you have been studying in vain for a decade or more, that you have been spending your days and nights at the hospital and missing out on "real life." Well, remember that the Lord Almighty knows your sacrifice to help others. At the perfect time, God will show up and you will see that the Lord will provide. And God will bless you far beyond what you imagine.

> *Then Abraham lifted his eyes and looked, and there behind him was a ram caught in a thicket by its horns... And Abraham called the name of the place, The-Lord-Will-Provide.*
>
> Genesis 22:13-14

> *By Myself I have sworn, says the Lord, because you have done this thing, and have*

> *not withheld your son, your only son - blessing I will bless you, and multiplying I will multiply your descendants as the stars of the heaven and as the sand which is on the seashore.*
>
> Genesis 22:16-17

God is looking for obedience. He delights in an obedient heart that says, "Lord, because You have said so, I will do it."

> *But Simon answered and said to Him, "Master, we have toiled all night and caught nothing; <u>nevertheless at Your word I will let down the net.</u>"*
>
> Luke 5:5 (emphasis added)

4. Take The Burden Of God's Kingdom

> *Come to Me, all you who labor and are heavy laden, and I will give you rest.*
>
> Matthew 11:28

> *Casting all your care upon Him, for He cares for you.*
>
> 1 Peter 5:7

In Matthew 11:30, Jesus says "My yoke is easy and My burden is light." The only true burden that we should be under is that of the Kingdom of God. I will put all other burdens at the cross and gladly pick up the yoke of Jesus.

> *Stand fast therefore in the liberty by which Christ has made us free, and do not be entangled again with a yoke of bondage.*
>
> Galatians 5:1

The Bible tells us to seek first the Kingdom of God (ref. Matthew 6:33) but the Bible doesn't name the second, third or fourth things to seek after that. That's because there are no second, third or fourth things. When I seek the Kingdom of God, I am seeking it with my family, friends, coworkers, patients, neighbors and associates. There is no division between serving God and living life. When I recognize who my King is and who I am in Christ, I have no excuse to live a half-hearted kingdom life at church on Sundays and a half-hearted worldly life during the week. The Kingdom of God is righteousness, peace, and joy in the Holy Spirit, all day everyday (ref. Romans 14:17).

In my daily life, whatever I am doing and wherever I am, I have worship songs or sermons playing in the background. Given that I am made of spirit, soul and body, I never want my spirit to be quiet during work time, study time, workout time, etc. While my soul and body are working on other things, my spirit is growing, praising the Lord and getting closer to Him. I always thought that I cannot serve God other than in a ministry at church, going on mission trips, preaching or leading worship. However, the Lord shifted my point of view and showed me the truth.

When I finally understood that I will be serving the Lord through my job as a doctor and that my ministry is with my patients and coworkers, I began to think: *What about now? How will I be able to serve the Lord in these 10-15 years of studying?* I found myself talking about Jesus with friends, family and random people. I found myself interceding for specific people the Lord highlighted to me. I was listening to messages, reading books and spending time in worship. All of that was my ministry during that season, allowing God to grow me and shape me into who He created me to be.

Don't waste the waiting! Don't wait until you can serve God where He called you to. Work on yourself and grow during this season of waiting. Allow the Lord to shape your heart to become like His own heart. Remember, David and Joseph both had to wait years for their callings to happen (around 20 and 13 years, respectively) but during that time, they were proclaiming the goodness of the Lord and worshiping His Holy name. They were serving God in the small groups where they lived.

David served the Lord among his soldiers and showed them how to love their enemies. He spared Saul's life twice, saying: "The Lord forbid that I should do this thing to my master, the Lord's anointed." Joseph served the Lord in prison, and his closeness to God enabled him to interpret the dreams of the prisoners and finally Pharaoh's dreams.

Live wisely during your season of waiting. Our lives are too short to rely on the upcoming years and say: "Fifteen years from now, when I become a doctor, I will pray with my patients." From this moment, ask God how you can serve Him. It might be through intercession, as the Lord put on my heart to be doing, or any other ministry. Don't wait another minute. We can never know when our last day on earth will be. There is so much more to the life we are living. Our first assignment is to be ambassadors of Christ seeking His kingdom and righteousness.

One thing I find extremely important is my secret time with the Lord. It is so easy to cancel time with God because *He understands that I am busy*. Besides, canceling my time with a coworker or friend will be "rude," but God loves me enough to forgive me. Or so I thought. Then I realized that it is I who actually do not understand. I do not understand how much of His peace, love and breakthrough I lose every time I neglect entering into His presence. "In Him we live and move and have our being" (Acts 17:28). It is I who do not understand how madly in love He is with me, and how supernatural of a life He is promising me as I get closer to Him.

We are co-heirs with Christ.

> *The Spirit Himself bears witness with our spirit that we are children of God, and if children then heirs-heirs of God and joint heirs with Christ, if indeed we suffer with Him, that we may also be glorified together.*
>
> Romans 8:16-17

"Prayerlessness creates lack and it will take me into temptations I don't have grace for. I may resist the temptations, but prayerlessness created a battle I didn't need to fight." ~ Bill Johnson

Prayer is the key to unlocking the Kingdom here on earth. No matter what comes or goes, as children of God, we need to clothe ourselves with the boldness of the Kingdom, knowing that Our Father is faithful to keep His promises. Our part is to bring Heaven to earth and to blindly trust God.

PRAYER

> *The Lord alone is our radiant hope and we trust in him with all our hearts. His wrap-around presence will strengthen us. As we trust, we rejoice with an uncontained joy flowing from Yahweh! Let your love and steadfast kindness overshadow us continually, for we trust and we wait upon you!*
>
> Psalm 33:20-22 TPT

Lord, I praise Your name and I glorify You because You are the One true God! You are Elohim and You created us to love us and to call us Your children. I come before You today and I make a covenant with You that, with the same trust I committed my life to Jesus and believed that eternal life is mine through faith in Him, I will trust You God with everything. You are faithful. You are the good Father! Amen!

5

Becoming Successful

In the supernatural environment of the Kingdom of God, success is defined differently than in the world. That is because God looks at the heart. For a child of God to be successful, they need only to obey His words and trust Him. King David was the man after God's own heart, and his son Solomon was the richest man to ever walk on earth. Before David died, he imparted a key to prosperity to his son.

> *And keep the charge of the Lord your God: to walk in His ways, to keep His statutes, His commandments, His judgments, and His testimonies, as it is written in the Law of Moses, that you may prosper in all that you do and wherever you turn.*
>
> 1 Kings 2:3

Notice how this diverges from conventional wisdom. The emphasis is on God, not self.

1. GOD'S LOVE IS BETTER THAN LIFE

> *Because <u>your love</u> is better than <u>life</u>, my lips will glorify you.*
>
> Psalm 63:3 NIV (emphasis added)

In the context of our discussion, I would like to explain this verse as such:

<u>Your love:</u>

> *God redeemed me; I am His child.*
> *God cares for me more than I care for myself.*
> *God has great things in store for me.*

<u>Life:</u>

> *My plans for myself.*
> *My vision of success.*

Jesus, Your name is *Love*. I praise You for who You are—the absolute definition of *Love*.

GOD REDEEMED ME AND CALLED ME HIS CHILD

> *For he who touches you touches the apple of His eye.*
>
> Zechariah 2:8

I always thought that sin was things like lying, stealing, sexual immorality, etc. However, I have come to understand that every single thing that breaks Jesus' heart is considered a sin. This was clear to me the moment I became aware of who I actually am in God's eyes compared to the way I talk to myself.

Every time you diminish yourself, curse yourself or speak negative things to yourself and about yourself, you are breaking Jesus' heart. Remember, you are the apple of His eye. You mean the world to Him. Wherever He is looking, you are at the center of His visual field. His mind is constantly overflowing with thoughts of you, His precious child. He called you by your name. You are His.

> *But now, thus says the Lord,*
> *Who created you, O Jacob,*
> *And He who formed you, O Israel:*
> *"Fear not, for I have redeemed you;*
> *I have called you by your name;*
> *You are Mine.*

Isaiah 43:1

I am the type of person who spends hours thinking, sometimes negatively. I used to dwell on the mistakes I'd made, my failures and the mountains yet to come.

I finally understood that entertaining bad thoughts and feeding your past failures are also sins in the sense that such behaviors are a departure from the nature of God. They neglect God's purpose and His perfect will for my life—the life that He established before I was even conceived.

> *Your eyes saw my substance, being yet unformed.*
> *And in Your book they all were written,*
> *The days fashioned for me,*
> *When as yet there were none of them.*
>
> Psalm 139:16

> *In Him also we have obtained an inheritance, being predestined according to the purpose of Him who works all things according to the counsel of His will,*
>
> Ephesians 1:11

Imagine if your best friend always talked negatively about your spouse. Wouldn't you question if they were truly your friend? Would you keep them in your life? Of course not. So, why are you entertaining curses spoken over your life? Why are you accepting them and feeding them? This breaks God's heart because He knows who He created you to be. He knows the real you that not even you have met yet. Talking yourself out of His calling means telling God "You are not telling the truth; I don't trust You enough. I am doing it my way."

"We ask ourselves, 'Who am I to be brilliant, gorgeous, talented, fabulous?' Actually, who are you not to be? You are a child of God." ~ Marianne Williamson

In our lives, we should only water the good trees that produce good fruits. We should uproot the poisonous trees and thorn bushes. Prophesy life over your future. Declare that you are God's. Seek His face day and night and expect an open heaven.

Every morning, declare peace, health, success, wealth and generational blessings to flow in you and through you! Speaking positively about yourself and encouraging yourself in the Lord are forms of worship and praise that bring glory to Him because He is the God of breakthrough.

O Lord, teach us how to let our lives and every breath we take glorify Your Holy name!

> *I bless you every time I take a breath.*
>
> Psalm 63:4, MSG

When I find it hard to forgive myself, I hear God's gentle voice whispering, "Peace unto you! I have forgiven you. Now it is your turn to forgive yourself and live the life I have set for you before you were even conceived."

God Cares For Me More Than I Care For Myself

Because God loves me more than I love myself, God cares for me more than I care for myself. I find myself praying: Forgive me Jesus when I think Your plans are so big that they are a burden. Forgive me when I flee from Your plans and reject them. Forgive me when I stick to my small dreams and ignore the resurrection power of the Holy Spirit living inside of me.

> *Trust in the Lord with all your heart, and lean not on your own understanding; in all your ways acknowledge Him, and He shall direct your paths.*
>
> Proverbs 3:5-6

We won't always know the answer to every question, but we know Jesus as *the answer*. If you want to know the "why" behind everything and spend your life trying to figure everything out, you are never going to find contentment. You will not enter the rest of God because trust always requires living with unanswered questions. We have to accept the unknown and be satisfied. We have to come to a place in our walk with God, where even though something doesn't seem fair or right, we love and trust God enough to know that He is still in control. He is working everything out for our good. Yes, we will have questions, but instead of lingering over them, God delights in hearing "I trust You."

> *And those who know Your name will put their trust in You; for You, Lord, have not forsaken those who seek You.*
>
> Psalm 9:10

It doesn't matter who tries to disqualify you. You have the most powerful force in you, the one and only living God who qualified you for a perfect calling.

> *For all the promises of God in Him are Yes, and in Him Amen, to the glory of God through us.*
>
> 2 Corinthians 1:20
>
> *God's gifts and God's call are under full warranty—never canceled, never rescinded.*
>
> Romans 11:29 MSG

Prayer

Father, when all is said and done, I will look back at what I have achieved and realize that You were holding me all along. It was not by my strength, nor by my power, but by Your Holy Spirit living in me. Your Power has given me this supernatural favor and success.

> *But we have this treasure in jars of clay to show that this all-surpassing power is from God and not from us.*
>
> 2 Corinthians 4:7 NIV

God Has Stored Great Things For Me

> *For I know the thoughts that I think toward you, says the Lord, thoughts of peace and not of evil, to give you a future and a hope.*
>
> Jeremiah 29:11

The plans of God for my life are already in place and have been there way before my birth. By Your unfailing love, Jesus, You have set the best for my life. You want me to succeed. You have already planned for me the brightest and most successful future that I could never attain without Your love.

> *Eye has not seen, nor ear heard, nor have entered into the heart of man the things which God has prepared for those who love Him.*
>
> 1 Corinthians 2:9

I dedicate my life to be the proof of God's goodness, mercy, blessings and grace. His innumerable promises are as clear as day. Even in the midst of trouble, God is The Good Father who protects me from all evil. Consider the scriptural evidence:

In the middle of the storm (the disciples).
In the lions' den (Daniel).
In the pit (Joseph).
In the hardships (Job).
Let the Prince of Peace comfort you.
Let Him speak life to you as you worship and praise His Holy name because He alone is worthy.

> *The Lord is my rock and my fortress and my deliverer; my God, my strength, in whom I will trust; my shield and the horn of my salvation, my stronghold. I will call upon the Lord, who is worthy to be praised*
>
> Psalm 18:2-3

PRAYER

Forgive me Jesus when I think I care more about my life than You do. Forgive me for settling with small dreams and thinking I will have great success by my own strength, for my own glory. All the glory belongs to You Jesus! You deserve it all!

> *Blessed is the man who trusts in the Lord, and whose hope is the Lord. For he shall be like a tree planted by the waters, which spreads out its roots by the river, and will not fear when heat comes; but its leaf will be green, and will not be anxious in the year of drought, nor will cease from yielding fruit.*
>
> Jeremiah 17:7-8

2. GETTING CLOSER TO JESUS

Understanding Jesus' love for me and getting closer to Him unlock heavenly blessings that carry my success. Getting closer means daily growth in the Word, worship, praise and intimacy. Jesus eagerly awaits to spend time with us. That is how much He loves us. That is why He created us.

By getting closer to God, He opens His heart to me and shows me His secrets.

> *Call to Me, and I will answer you, and show you great and mighty things, which you do not know.*
>
> Jeremiah 33:3

> *There's a private place reserved for the lovers of God, where they sit near Him and receive the revelation-secrets of His promises.*
>
> Psalm 25:14 TPT

We are called to be creative, just as the Father is. He created the whole universe, and created the human being in all his complexity. I want to be as creative as my Father. I want to spend time in His presence and learn from Him the secrets to becoming creative—new inventions, new ideas, new art, new medical treatment. If the world has the wisdom to innovate, how much more should we explore new horizons. As God's children, we have access to God's perfect wisdom.

> *If any of you lacks wisdom, let him ask of God, who gives to all liberally and without reproach, and it will be given to him.*
>
> James 1:5

> *Because the foolishness of God is wiser than men, and the weakness of God is stronger than men.*
>
> 1 Corinthians 1:25

God is perfect in knowledge. He created all things and will reveal them to us as we seek Him and ask Him. He delights in seeing His children prosper. It takes us one leap of faith to dare to ask God for wisdom concerning our studies, how to deal with others, how to create novel treatment, etc. After all, He created the universe and He knows how everything works in the finest details. Every single thing in this world was already God's created idea. We just discover them.

If I asked God for wisdom regarding some human discovery, would He say, "Oh wait a minute! Let me check the manual. I don't know how this works"? Of course not! He is the Creator of everything. He is the All-knowing God. He is Omniscient. Nothing takes Him by surprise. He knows all that can be known and all there is to know.

> *All things were made through Him, and without Him nothing was made that was made.*
>
> John 1:3

Prosperity and success are biblical terms. As such, they have different meanings than the worldly definitions. According to the Bible, as long as I seek the Lord, I am prosperous.

When asked about the greatest commandment, Jesus replied: "You shall love the Lord your God with all your heart, with all your soul, and with all your mind" (Matthew 22:37). When I learn to truly give my all to God, He will reward me with abundant blessings.

> *Blessed is the man... his delight is in the law of the Lord, and in His law meditates day and night. He shall be like a tree planted by the rivers of water, that brings forth its fruit in its season, whose leaf also shall not wither; and whatever he does prosper.*
>
> Psalm 1:1-3

> *David continued to succeed in everything he did, for the Lord was with him.*
>
> 1 Samuel 18:14 NLT

God gives us the tools to succeed but it is our responsibility to make it happen. It is not easy to take time in prayer and sit in the presence of the Lord every day. Seeking God and meditating on His Word day and night requires sacrifice. I am sacrificing the priorities that the world has set for me in order to give myself to Jesus. Every time I sit in the presence of God, I get a deeper understanding of how amazing He is. I learn a new nature of Him, and this grows my reverential fear towards Him—the most amazing type of fear.

> *He sought God during the days of Zechariah, who instructed him in the fear of God. As long as he sought the Lord, God gave him success.*
>
> 2 Chronicles 26:5 NIV
>
> *The fear of the Lord is the beginning of wisdom, and the knowledge of the Holy One is understanding.*
>
> Proverbs 9:10

The fear of God is the knowledge of His sovereignty and the countless expressions of His nature, coupled with the knowledge that He gave everything to die for my sins and to redeem me to His Kingdom. How can I not sacrifice my entire life to live for such a King? What responsibility is greater than taking time to glorify my Lord and King?

Success comes when my identity in Christ becomes carved in me just as my name is engraved on the palms of God's hands.

> *See, I have inscribed you on the palms of My hands.*
>
> Isaiah 49:16

Then I understand that I am a victor, not a victim. I am righteous because of the cross. I am the head and not the tail. The triumphant Lion of the tribe of Judah lives in me.

> *Yet in all these things we are more than conquerors through Him who loved us.*
>
> Romans 8:37

I am responsible for my own prosperity and my own success by embracing my identity as a Christian. God wants me to excel, and through Him, I will. Rather...*we* will, He and I, together.

> *But Moses said to God, "Who am I that I should go to Pharaoh, and that I should bring the children of Israel out of Egypt?" ... And God said to Moses, "I AM WHO I AM." And He said, "Thus you shall say to the children of Israel, 'I AM has sent me to you.'"*
>
> Exodus 3:11, 14

We should learn to reply to our circumstances just like God answered Moses. If my critics say "You are not enough, you can't do this on your own," I will reply, "I am who Jesus says I am because He is who He says He is."

As sons and daughters, God has given us divine favor. Consider the summation of God's commandments to the fledgling nation of the children of Israel by their leader, Moses.

> *Now it shall come to pass, if you diligently obey the voice of the Lord your God, to observe carefully all His commandments which I command you today, that the Lord your God will set you high above all nations of the earth. And all these blessings shall come upon you and overtake you, because you obey the voice of the Lord your God.*
>
> Deuteronomy 28:1-2

Notice that in verses 3 to 13, Moses proclaims blessings in different areas of life: the dwelling place, the family, the work, the food, and the myriad paths and byways that the journey in life will take them to.

The enemy has no power over you. Everything you put in your hand will prosper and come to maturity. You will find favor with every person you meet. You will lend and not borrow. You will rise to the top, not sink to the bottom.

Yet all these promises come with a cost. Notice the qualifying statement: "If you keep the commands of the Lord your God and walk in obedience to him". Our Father has great riches stored for each of us, and He delights in giving His children gifts. But He is waiting on our obedience. This is how a good father trains his children to walk in righteousness.

"The Lord wants to raise a generation of people who will learn to live from the presence of God as opposed to merely living from the principles of God. And that's a big deal because with the principles, there is success but with the Presence, there is no failure." ~ Bill Johnson

PRAYER

Lord, forgive our laziness and unbelief. We blame the world and our responsibilities for not spending time in your presence, but everything comes back to our choices. Today, we choose to host Your presence. We choose to carry the very atmosphere of heaven wherever we go. We want to see Your promises in our lives. Let Your will be done in our lives as it is in heaven! Amen!

> *For the Lord God is a sun and shield; the Lord will give grace and glory; no good thing will He withhold from those who walk uprightly. O Lord of hosts, blessed is the man who trusts in You.*
>
> Psalm 84:11-12

3. Run Your Own Race

Everyone has a goal, a dream, a drive for running. Let each of us run our own race at our own pace. We are all in this together, as a team. Each of us is an element and we are supposed to be there for each other.

I love what the great woman of God, Lisa Bevere, wrote in her book *Without Rival*.

"I heard the Holy Spirit whisper, 'I do not love my children equally... Equal implies my love can be measured, and I assure you... it cannot. Same would mean my children are replaceable or interchangeable, and they are not. My heart is not divided into compartments. No one could take the place of or displace another in my heart. For you see, I don't love my children equally, I love them uniquely."

We are to embrace the unique love of Christ for each of us, seeking to encourage one another and lift each other up. Every person has a unique path in life. Even if there are thousands of doctors from the same specialty, each one has a different calling in life. I will not treat the same patients as my colleagues. I will not work with the same coworkers as my colleagues. I will have other projects to work on. All things are pre-designed by God to cross my unique journey in life. And the Lord is waiting to see how I will react to these challenges and adventures.

God has a river of blessings for each and every one of us. He does not withhold any good thing from us. The flow never stops, but we have to reach out and grab blessings from it. As long as we trust God and know our position in Christ, and as long as we approach the living waters, we will be blessed.

> *He who did not spare His own Son, but delivered Him up for us all, how shall He not with Him also freely give us all things?*
>
> Romans 8:32

Receive His love. Be bold to reach out and grab your blessings from your river. It's your river, not someone else's. God wrote your beginning and end. He knows every detail you will need. He did not forget a thing, so do not search for blessings elsewhere.

My strength comes from knowing that I am saved by God's grace. I am God's child. It should not depend on whether or not I am good enough, intelligent enough, or at the top of my field. Comparison is the worst thing we can inflict upon ourselves. Nothing good comes from it. Comparison steals our peace, joy and identity.

Let's look at how it worked out for Moses.

> *Then Moses said to the Lord, "O my Lord, I am not eloquent, neither before nor since You have spoken to Your servant; but I am slow to speech and slow of tongue." So the Lord said to him, "Who has made man's mouth? Or who makes the mute, the deaf, the seeing, or the blind? Have not I, the Lord? Now therefore, go, and I will be with your mouth and teach you what you shall say." But he said, "O my Lord, please send by the hand of whomever else You may send."*
>
> Exodus 4:10-13

Have you ever wondered what would have happened if Moses hadn't said this last sentence? Would God have helped him as He promised: "I will be with your mouth and teach you what you shall say" (verse 12)? Our problem is that we think God is going to take us to the mountain peaks and abandon us there. Yes, betrayal is the major cause of our doubts, but it happens because of people, not God. We should never assign our doubts and fears to God.

The worst thing you can do to yourself is to question God and doubt what He tells you. Don't ponder, just obey! On several occasions during my medical training, the Lord asked me to pray for specific patients. During those moments, hundreds of thoughts crossed my mind, and I gave God many arguments to convince Him why it would be better to not pray for the sick, and why it would be better to send someone else.

I thank God He didn't listen to me! By His abundant mercy, He kept the fire burning within me until I obeyed and prayed for them. Never let your reasoning logic be stronger than the Holy Spirit burning within you.

Be ready to say "Yes" the moment God calls you to a journey of destiny. Never say "No." It only delays the inevitable. Don't tell God to send someone else, and don't try to run away from God as Jonah did. The King of kings is sending you specifically for a precise purpose. Just trust and obey Him. He is your Father and He wants the best for you. He delights in seeing you grow and trusting His word. He will never leave you halfway through your journey. He will never let you down. At the end of the road, you will be surprised by what you accomplished and how the Lord cheered you all the way through it.

> *And He said to me, "My grace is sufficient for you, for My strength is made perfect in weakness."*
>
> 2 Corinthians 12:9
>
> *And let us run with endurance the race that is set before us, looking unto Jesus, the author and finisher of our faith.*
>
> Hebrews 12:1-2

4. WE ARE SPECIAL

People always ask me, "What do you do outside of studying/working?"

I reply, "I go to church two to three days a week."

Then I get a weird response as if I am "so boring."

One day, the Lord spoke to me. "You are special. There's nothing wrong with being special."

I knew it was about His calling on my life, about being a doctor in His image. I knew it was related to my walk with the Lord and how I love to go to church and spend time in prayer. This is the most valuable part of my life. Jesus is my all, and confirming to me that it is not wrong to be special pushes me to pursue Him even more, to pray bolder prayers, to accept criticism and persecution. God gave me His all, and He deserves my all. Few are the people who follow Jesus and walk through the narrow path. I choose to be one of those few.

> *Enter by the narrow gate; for wide is the gate and broad is the way that leads to destruction, and there are many who go in by it. Because narrow is the gate and difficult is the way which leads to life, and there are few who find it.*
>
> Matthew 7:13-14

Life can be a tough competition. In an environment where everyone tries to outdo the other, it can be hard to find a faithful friend who rejoices in your success and strengthens you when you are down. But Christians have the most faithful friend. He is Immanuel—*God with us*. He is our biggest fan. We should be learning from Him this priceless character of being a faithful friend.

> *Whoever refreshes others will be refreshed.*
>
> Proverbs 11:25 NIV

As I said earlier, there is a spiritual river flowing for every person. You don't have to look into your neighbor's river and try to catch their blessings. You have your own river where God overflows His special blessings for your life.

> *Now to Him who is able to do exceedingly abundantly above all that we ask or think, according to the power that works in us.*
>
> Ephesians 3:20

> *"For My thoughts are not your thoughts, nor are your ways My ways," says the Lord. "For as the heavens are higher than the earth, so*

are My ways higher than your ways and My thoughts than your thoughts."

Isaiah 55:8-9

As doctors, we endure hardships in medical school and residency. We suffer loneliness, fatigue and burnout. We know how it feels to be anxious or criticized. Let us be careful with what we say to others and be careful with what we say to ourselves. As much as you need encouragement, people need to hear uplifting words. Before saying anything, always practice the words in your mind as if they were directed to you. Don't say anything that you would not accept being said about you.

Let us learn from Jesus how to love unconditionally, especially how to love ourselves, because the moment we appreciate that truth, we will have a bigger assignment—to love our neighbors as ourselves.

Until then, there are three things that remain: faith, hope, and love – yet love surpasses them all. So above all else, let love be the beautiful prize for which you run.

1 Corinthians 13:13 TPT

Prayer

Our Heavenly Father, we thank You for Your unfailing and unconditional Love. Thank You for making us Your righteousness through Your Holy son Jesus Christ and His work on the cross. It is finished! The cross is the final and perfect work. It is the seal that brought us back to You. We delight in You and choose to follow You because of who You are and what You have done. Teach us to love ourselves and give us the wisdom and courage to treat others as Your sons and daughters, and to love them as we love ourselves. Help us not to seek the blessings but rather to seek Your face, O Lord! And as we seek Your face, Your abundant promises will come to pass, for You are faithful and true. We are eternally thankful to You.

6

Work-Life Balance

Are you tired? Worn out? Burned out on religion? Come to me. Get away with me and you'll recover your life. I'll show you how to take a real rest. Walk with me and work with me – watch how I do it. Learn the unforced rhythms of grace. I won't lay anything heavy or ill-fitting on you. Keep company with me and you'll learn to live freely and lightly.

Matthew 11:28-30 MSG

1. REST IN GOD

And He said, "My Presence will go with you, and I will give you rest."

Exodus 33:14

Truly my soul finds rest in God; my salvation comes from him.

Psalm 62:1 NIV

God entrusted me with my personal life as much as He entrusted me with my work life. He would never want me to stop caring about myself. This is not healthy and was never meant to be part of a doctor's life. The Lord wants to see if I am able to wisely manage my time—giving my best to study hard but never ignoring my body, soul and spirit.

Here is how I care for myself.

My soul:

- reading the Bible
- praying
- worshiping
- allowing God to work on me and through me

My spirit:

- spending time with family and friends
- choosing the right people whose relationships are healthy for growth
- eliminating toxic relationships
- spending time reflecting on life
- planning for the future

My body:

- eating healthy
- exercising
- relaxing
- having fun

I'm not saying it's always easy, but it's manageable. At first, I was awful at managing my life, but as I persevered, the Lord saw my efforts and guided my small steps. I may never perfect it. In fact, it is God's part to touch the end result, to refine and perfect the big picture. However, God expects me to be faithful in the little He has given me. He is waiting for me to present Him my part of the work, then He will do His part of purification. He delights in the baby steps I take to change my life toward the best. I desire to hear Him say, "Well done, good and faithful servant; you have been faithful over a few things, I will make you ruler over many things. Enter into the joy of your lord" (Matthew 25:23).

During medical school, I found it difficult to take time for myself. My only excuse was "I have so much to study for. I want to be successful. There is no time for fun."

As the weight of studies grew heavier, I began to dedicate time every day to listening to motivational speakers talk about how to keep pressing on, how to give 120%, how to wake up before everyone else because there was no time to lose in order to be great.

Unfortunately, these motivational speeches turned out to be a double-edged sword for me. They were perfect poison. Let me explain.

Motivation is great for a person who procrastinates or who has trouble moving forward. But I find that it can be quite destructive in a person who is already hustling and *needs* to take a break and learn to enjoy life. I used to always say to myself, "I can study without taking any break. I am strong. I can survive this." And indeed, I did survive several years, but I crashed hard afterwards. During that period, I received a word from the Lord telling me to take care of my body. I was adamant, however, that I could manage myself just fine without obeying God's word. That was right before I nosedived into burnout and depression.

What I learned from this experience was that the Bible is the perfect place to draw inspiration, motivation, and life coaching. *The Bible is the manual that comes with you in order to understand how to function in life.* It is the living Word of God, full of wisdom and power.

In this context, I would like to highlight a few verses from one of the books of wisdom:

> *To everything there is a season, a time for every purpose under heaven.*
>
> Ecclesiastes 3:1

> *What profit has the worker from that in which he labors? I have seen the God-given task with which the sons of men are to be occupied. He has made everything beautiful in its time. Also He has put eternity in their hearts, except that no one can find out the work that God does from beginning to end. I know that nothing is better for them than to rejoice, and to do good in their lives, and also that every man should eat and drink and enjoy the good of all his labor - it is the gift of God.*
>
> Ecclesiastes 3: 9-13

In life, there is a time for everything. The Lord says: "While the earth remains, seedtime and harvest shall not cease" (Genesis 8:22). Yet between these two seasons there is always time to rest. And this law is true for any kind of labor. We put forth the effort required from us and then we rest and wait for our victory which comes from God.

> *Unless the Lord builds the house, they labor in vain who build it.*
>
> Psalm 127:1
>
> *You can do your best to prepare for the battle, but ultimate victory comes from the Lord God.*
>
> Proverbs 21:31 TPT
>
> *Before you do anything, put your trust totally in God and not in yourself. Then every plan you make will succeed.*
>
> Proverbs 16:3 TPT

This is not meant to be an invitation to be lazy. On the contrary, the Bible talks a lot about productivity and how a wise person values hard work.

> *He who has a slack hand becomes poor, but the hand of the diligent makes rich.*
>
> Proverbs 10:4
>
> *In all labor there is profit, but idle chatter leads only to poverty.*
>
> Proverbs 14:23

He who tills his land will be satisfied with bread, but he who follows frivolity is devoid of understanding.

Proverbs 12:11

One thing I have learned the hard way is that when I get tired, I should slow down and rest. Sounds simple, right? Except when you are driven to excel, rest is the enemy. The balance is that getting tired should never be a reason to quit. It is merely to take a break, rejuvenate and remember why you're trying so hard in the first place.

Every person has a different way of resting. During my breaks, I love to listen to worship songs, sermons or audiobooks while working out. I find this much more revitalizing than watching TV or going to the mall. When I go out, I almost always go to church or a prayer meeting because this is where I find rest and joy. Other people enjoy the movies or a restaurant with friends. We are all different, so don't feel obliged to spend your free time as others do. You may like different activities than most people. That's normal. I sometimes hear: *You're boring; you're too religious; you gotta loosen up.* And this is from people who love me! The key is to do what you like. Do what you know pleases God and draws you closer to Him.

2. Rest Is A Gift

What better example to be set before us than the creation of the world—no small feat—and how God dedicated a day to rest.

> *And on the seventh day God ended His work which He had done, and He rested on the seventh day.*
>
> Genesis 2:2

I am sure God never gets tired. He is God, of course! With a few words He created the entire universe! But I believe this verse was written as an example for us to follow. If the God of the universe took time to rest and gaze at the beauty He had created, how much more do we need to rest and enjoy the labor of six days?

> *Six days you shall work, but on the seventh day you shall rest; in plowing time and in harvest you shall rest.*
>
> Exodus 34:21

We were created in God's image, so our bodies, souls and spirits need to rest just as He rested. One of the things I regret the most in my life is not listening to my loved ones who were constantly telling me to take a break.

Ever since I was young, I was always told "You are so intelligent and brave. I wish I could study like you and get good grades like you do." This was a huge motivation to study harder and move forward. I thought my ability to stay in my room for hours and study was the thing that made me so special and clever. I kept repeating what people said about me. I fed on their words, and every year, I kept myself in my room studying longer. Little did I know that these encouraging words would turn out to be my biggest enemy.

My close family noticed the toxic path I had been dragged into. They constantly told me to forget my studies for a few hours every week and take a break. All I'd say was, "I have a lot of studies. I don't have time for a break. After all, even if I go out, I won't enjoy my time because all I would think of are my studies."

What a lie! I was entangled in a vicious cycle. I knew something was wrong, but I was too submerged in the toxic thoughts I used to drive myself. The situation became hopeless. In my darkest moments, I begged God to change His calling over my life, to give me an easy job so I could enjoy my life.

The truth is, any job is easy when it is what God calls us to. I'm not saying it's not hard work, but the work is a joy... when the joy of the Lord is our strength.

> *Here is what I have seen: It is good and fitting for one to eat and drink, and to enjoy the good of all his labor in which he toils under the sun all the days of his life which God gives him; for it is his heritage. As for every man to whom God has given riches and wealth, and given him power to eat of it, to receive his heritage and rejoice in his labor - this is the gift of God. For he will not dwell unduly on the days of his life, because God keeps him busy with the joy of his heart.*
>
> Ecclesiastes 5:18-20

As much as it is a blessing to work, be productive and earn money, rest is a gift from God. I want to follow the example of my Heavenly Father who rested on the seventh day. God saw that everything He created was good, and He took a day off to enjoy it. I want to enjoy the fruit of my labor now, daily and weekly, instead of counting the number of years I have before graduation or retirement. Rest is part of God's plan.

I want my heart to be occupied with such happiness that I forget how hard life can be. I want to enjoy every moment of my life whether it is hard work or rest time. God will take care of the details just as He did when He carefully formed me in my mother's womb.

> *It really is senseless to work so hard from early morning till late at night, toiling to make a living for fear of not having enough. God can provide for his lovers even while they sleep!*
>
> Psalm 127:2 TPT

Work will become enjoyable as we seek God's kingdom, drawing closer to Jesus in all we do. This is because we will do our work as for the Lord, which leads us to a new realm where:

Strength is drawn from our identity in Christ.

> *For the joy of the Lord is your strength.*
>
> Nehemiah 8:10

Peace overflows from the Prince of Peace.

> *And the peace of God, which surpasses all understanding, will guard your hearts and minds through Christ Jesus.*
>
> Philippians 4:7

Goodness and mercy follow us everywhere.

> *Surely goodness and mercy shall follow me all the days of my life; and I will dwell in the house of the Lord forever.*
>
> Psalm 23:6

A believer's guide to success and abundance lies in inviting Jesus into their boat.

> *Now when evening came, His disciples went down to the sea, got into the boat, and went over the sea toward Capernaum. And it was already dark, and Jesus had not come to them. Then the sea arose because a great wind was blowing. So when they had rowed about three or four miles, they saw Jesus walking on the sea and drawing near the boat; and they were afraid. But He said to them, "It is I; do not be afraid." Then they willingly received Him into the boat, and immediately the boat was at the land where they were going.*
>
> John 6:16-21

Through perfect circumstances and storms, I know that God is in control. His joy, peace and mercy fill my boat.

3. GLORY TO GLORY

How can I grow from glory to glory? How can my life and family be blessed? It all depends on what I do with what God has given me.

> *For whoever has, to him more will be given, and he will have abundance; but whoever does not have, even what he has will be taken away from him.*
>
> Matthew 13:12

Remember the widow at the time of Elijah. She thought she had nothing, but the little she had saved her life and her son's life until the famine had passed.

> *So she said, "As the Lord your God lives, I do not have bread, only a handful of flour in a bin, and a little oil in a jar; and see, I am gathering a couple of sticks that I may go in and prepare it for myself and my son, that we may eat it, and die.*
>
> 1 King 17:12

Remember the five loaves and two fish that satisfied the hunger of 5,000 men, besides women and children, in John 6? If that little boy had not given his lunch to Jesus, they would have never eaten, nor would they have witnessed a miracle. The meal lasted a day; the miracle has lasted for 2,000 years.

It is not my job to multiply, only to give. I just have to be faithful in handing God the resources I have, then trust and believe that He is the miracle maker, the One who takes the impossibilities and turns them into a supernatural flow of blessings for me and my surroundings.

Here are some important steps to take to grow from glory to glory:

1. Pursue intimacy with God: seek Him for growth.
2. Fellowship with family, friends and church: iron sharpens iron.
3. Pour into others: foster the growth of my patients and coworkers.

My Time With God

We are all invited to pursue intimacy with God. Our daily time with God should be our top priority. I spend time in God's presence, talking to Him, worshiping Him and allowing His gentle voice to speak life over me. In reading the Bible, I grow deeper in God's knowledge and wisdom. In order to be successful, I have learned to fully preoccupy myself with God's Kingdom.

> *Delight yourself also in the Lord, and He shall give you the desires of your heart.*
>
> Psalm 37:4
>
> *For the Lord takes delight in his people; he crowns the humble with victory.*
>
> Psalm 149:4 NIV

When my faith is strong, I feel that I am so close to Jesus that I will never miss His presence no matter what. This is a fallacy, however. When my faith is strong, it is then that I have to keep feeding it. Faith is like a fire. The day I don't fuel it is the day it recedes and cools. God promised to never leave us. Yet it is the awareness of His presence that we are seeking.

Be alerted to the day you consider your faith is stronger than a mustard seed. The strength that you are experiencing is only found in God's presence, as you walk together with Him. As soon as you step out of His presence, your weakness will be revealed.

> *This Book of the Law shall not depart from your mouth, but you shall meditate in it day and night, that you may observe to do*

> *according to all that is written in it. For then you will make your way prosperous, and then you will have good success.*
>
> Joshua 1:8

Always remember that you can barely climb few steps without God. Then you will stagnate at the same place or fall down the stairs. When God's hand is not holding your back, you are vulnerable to a fall. Thank God for His discipleship and constant help. Nothing feels better than His hand on your back, pushing you forward and steadying you lest you fall.

> *The LORD makes firm the steps of the one who delights in him; though he may stumble, he will not fall, for the LORD upholds him with his hand.*
>
> Psalm 37:23-24 NIV

PRAYER

Oh Lord, forgive me when I get to a place of contentment, when I consider myself strong enough to move on my own. The truth is, without you I am weak. Without Your presence, I am but fragile clay. Take my heart and refine me to become more like You. Teach me to rely on nothing but Your precious Word, the cornerstone, Jesus Christ. Holy are You Lord! Amen!

<u>MY TIME WITH MY LOVED ONES</u>

Spiritual growth comes not only by spending time with the Lord and reading the Word, but also by time spent with family and friends, including my church family.

> *As iron sharpens iron, so a man sharpens the countenance of his friend.*
>
> Proverbs 27:17

Hearing and sharing testimonies, praising God as a group, believing for a miracle together—these are a few of the examples that lead us to stronger faith. In this world, I was never meant to fight by myself. Jesus sent out His disciples two by two (ref. Mark 6:7). There is power in united faith.

> *Again I say to you that if two of you agree on earth concerning anything that they ask, it will be done for them by My Father in heaven. For where two or three are gathered together in My name, I am there in the midst of them."*
>
> Matthew 18:19-20

> *In him you too are being built together to become a dwelling in which God lives by his Spirit.*
>
> Ephesians 2:22 NIV

Work and studies will never end, so don't try to chase them every minute of the day. Learn to stop and ponder the beauty of life. Your parents need your help. Your children need your full attention. Your spouse is eager to spend time with you. Your body is begging you to treat it well.

Listen to the Holy Spirit and spend your days wisely. Life is not over; this is your opportunity to change.

> *So teach us to number our days, that we may gain a heart of wisdom.*
>
> Psalm 90:12

A few worship songs on our way home will not satisfy our hunger and thirst. I compare this to someone who has been waiting for summer so he can swim in the ocean. Yet as soon as he gets there, he dips his feet in the water and goes back home. Did he satisfy his winter's longing to swim in the ocean? Not even close!

Unfortunately, we do the same with our spiritual lives. We go to church for an hour on Sunday, we sing three worship songs, we listen to a 30-minute sermon and think that this "sip of water" will satisfy our thirst for the whole week. It won't.

How can I pour joy and faith into my kids, my spouse and my friends? How can I pour hope and strength into my patients and coworkers? We are supposed to be the light of the world. We are supposed to have "rivers of living water" flowing from us. The Lord alone is the source of all light and living water. To be able to carry them to the world, we must be immersed in His presence.

Expand your vessel every day and ask for more of His presence. A small bottle will only be enough for you alone. Get a gallon-size spiritual vessel and ask for more to be able to give away.

<u>My Time With My Patients/Coworkers</u>

As the peace of God fills my heart, I will be able to enjoy my work and the time I spend with my co-workers and patients. My divine assignment is to love them and to be Jesus' fragrance among them. I might be their only hope! By pouring into them, I help them grow spiritually as well.

When asked about how she prays for the sick to get healed, the great woman of God, Heidi Baker, replied:

"God spoke to me many times that my job is to love, and His job is to heal... Sometimes we're so interested in the end result that we forget the person along the way. It is about sharing compassion and love, then you can't fail because people leave feeling loved, and that's what matters."

> *Love never fails. But where there are prophecies, they will cease; where there are tongues, they will be stilled; where there is knowledge, it will pass. For we know in part and we prophesy in part, but when completeness comes, what is in part disappears.*
>
> 1 Corinthians 13:8-10 NIV

Where there is medicine and medical treatments, they will cease, but love remains. So, let us keep on loving the patients and praying for them, because even if our knowledge and medicine fail, we have given the patients our best, which is Christ in us, the Hope of the world. Remember: we do our best, and God perfects it.

We are working with people whom Christ loves and died for.

> *The King will reply, "Truly I tell you, whatever you did for one of the least of these brothers and sisters of mine, you did for me."*
>
> Matthew 25:40

4. Peace Through It All

> *You will keep him in perfect peace, whose mind is stayed on You, because he trusts in You. Trust in the Lord forever, for in YAH, the Lord, is everlasting strength.*
>
> Isaiah 26:3-4

God never promised us a life without problems. Instead, He promised that in the middle of the storms, we can have peace—the peace that transcends all understanding and protects us.

How is that possible? By action. You see, every time David experienced a hard time, he ordered his soul to be still. He made a commitment with his soul that they would not be shaken.

I always thought that peace was achieved by faith alone. Then I learned that peace is the substance of faith and mostly of work.

> *Be anxious for nothing, but in everything by prayer and supplication, with thanksgiving, let your requests be made known to God; and the peace of God which surpasses all understanding, will guard your hearts and minds through Christ Jesus.*
>
> Philippians 4:6-7

Every time I faced a problem, I used to pray "Lord, I believe You are the Prince of Peace. I ask that You fill my heart with Your abundant Peace." Then I stress about the situation and expect God to pour His perfect peace on me as if someone was pouring water over my head. This seldom happened, and I've since learned that this is not how peace usually works.

> *And which of you by worrying can add one cubit to his stature? If you then are not able to do the least, why are you anxious for the rest?*
>
> Luke 12:25-26

After I spend time in prayer and ask God for peace, I have to take time with myself and speak to my soul.

The decisions and commitments that we take with our souls play a big role in our Christian lives. By the same way we grow in our relationship with God through prayer, we grow our souls when we empower them with the right words.

- *Soul, trust in the Lord for He is good and His love endures forever.*
- *Soul, be still and know that God holds your future.*
- *Soul, you are deeply loved by the Lord Almighty, so get back on your feet.*

Return to your rest, O my soul, for the Lord has dealt bountifully with you.

Psalm 116:7

Why are you cast down, O my soul? And why are you disquieted within me? Hope in God; for I shall yet praise Him, the help of my countenance and my God.

Psalm 42:11

Be the coach of your soul. Acquire the habit of training your soul and you will see how your soul can find strength in the Lord. Remind your soul of what God has done for it. Remind your soul of who the Lord is and how glorious He is. Command it to bless the Lord.

If you train well your soul, it will acquire a quick reflex to turn its ear to you whenever it is shaken by a problem. You are your soul's coach. It will always listen to your words. So, let your words be full of life!

As we learn to be sensitive to our spiritual thirst and put God above all, we experience His deepest love for us.

> *That you, being rooted and grounded in love, may be able to comprehend with all the saints what is the width and length and depth and height - to know the love of Christ which passes knowledge; that you may be filled with all the fullness of God.*
>
> Ephesians 3:17-19

5. An Ounce Of Prevention

One of the most powerful aspects of medicine is prevention, especially primary prevention. We need to understand that the trouble we get into by not putting God first is *preventable.* Our major excuse is lack of time. Yet we spend a lot more time trying to fix our problems through our own strength than if we had never turned away from God in the first place.

Operating solely in our own strength produces stress and anxiety, shorter attention span with our patients, and deteriorating relationships with friends and family. We can avoid this waste of time, hope and energy by drawing near to God and maintaining our relationship with Him.

Prevention is key. There's no compromise. My time with the lover of my heart is priceless. It is my one and only, everlasting and overflowing treasure. How blessed are we to be sons and daughters of the Most High God!

> *Give God the right to direct your life, and as you trust him along the way you'll find he pulled it off perfectly!*
>
> Psalm 37:5 TPT

Conclusion

As you go through this journey, I would like to encourage you to seek what matters. Jesus is the source of all life, joy and success. Following His calling for your life is worth your sacrifice. The Bible clearly says that opposition will come but you already won through Christ our Savior. Run this race with Jesus and commit to seeking His Kingdom wherever you go.

You are not here by chance. You were called to be a doctor. You were called to make a difference in the medical community. You were called to follow the Great Physician.

> *Because of this, since I first heard about your strong faith in the Lord Jesus Christ and your tender love toward all his devoted ones, my heart is always full and overflowing with thanks to God for you as I constantly remember you in my prayers. I pray that the Father of glory, the God of our Lord Jesus Christ, would impart to you the riches of the Spirit of wisdom and the Spirit of revelation to know him through your deepening intimacy with him. I pray that the light of God will*

illuminate the eyes of your imagination, flooding you with light, until you experience the full revelation of the hope of his calling — that is, the wealth of God's glorious inheritances that he finds in us, his holy ones! I pray that you will continually experience the immeasurable greatness of God's power made available to you through faith. Then your lives will be an advertisement of this immense power as it works through you! This is the mighty power that was released when God raised Christ from the dead and exalted him to the place of highest honor and supreme authority in the heavenly realm! And now he is exalted as first above every ruler, authority, government, and realm of power in existence! He is gloriously enthroned over every name that is ever praised, not only in this age, but in the age that is coming!

Ephesians 1:15-21 TPT

Acknowledgements

To God the Father, the Son and the Holy Spirit – From the moment I said "Yes" to You, my life was drastically changed. I have known You as the glorious King and as the sweetest friend. You have been my ever-present help in every step of the way. I am living in constant breakthroughs because You are such a loving Father. My "Thank You" will never be enough. All I have to offer are my praise and my alabaster heart.

To Jim Bryson – You are blessed with natural editing skills. Thank you for the wonderful job you did. And thank you for your ongoing encouragement and humor, as they both empowered me to press on and publish my first book. It has been such an honor partnering with you. Thank you.

To Gary Williams – My personal coach from the Self-Publishing School. Thank you for keeping up with me as my journey took longer than expected. Still, becoming a published author is more rewarding than I could have ever imagined. Your help is deeply appreciated. Thank you.

To Joe Tannous – From all the interests we share, I never imagined writing books would be a common passion of ours. I am truly blessed by our priceless friendship. Thank you for always listening to me and offering genuine support. Thank you.

To Michelle Borckardt – Our friendship is a blessing to me. The way we met and the way we kept each other accountable through our writing journeys are a testimony that God preserves the best for the ones who love Him. Thank you.

To 100 Covers team – Thank you for the amazing book cover you provided to me. Working with you was a pleasure. Thank you.

About the Author

Since age five, Melissa's dream was to become a doctor. In 2017, she made her dream reality, graduating from Saint Joseph University in Beirut, Lebanon with a Doctor of Medicine degree. Melissa then moved to the U.S. to continue her medical training.

Melissa grew up in a Christian family, but she personally encountered Jesus at the age of fifteen. Shortly after, she received a prophetic word confirming her childhood dream of becoming a doctor. It was a life-changing experience when she became aware that her heart's desire was aligned with God's calling for her life. Melissa was then ready to start her journey, knowing that the Holy Spirit was guiding her steps.

As a medical student, Melissa experienced burnout and questioned the possibility of serving God through medicine. She then realized that there must be more to medicine than what is taught and practiced. Becoming a doctor is not merely a career choice. It is a true calling—a divine one that carries God's love, hope and power to the world. Empathy and medical care are not enough. They both are strong pillars in medicine; however, they should be driven by Christ-like love. Love that is unconditional.

As she fixes her eyes on Jesus, Melissa's goal is to become more like Him in every aspect of life. In her prayer time, she once heard the Lord say, "Tear down the boxes you have put me in and the boxes you have put yourself in, and watch what I'll do." Since then, Melissa is living in daily breakthroughs, allowing Jesus to reveal Himself to her and learning her place in God's heart.

Melissa can be reached here:
www.facebook.com/followingthegreatphysician
Followinggreatphysician@gmail.com

Can You Help?

Thank You for Reading My Book!

I really appreciate all of your feedback, and I love hearing what you have to say.

Please leave an **honest review on Amazon** letting me know what you thought of the book and how it impacted your life.

Thank you so much!

~ Melissa Khalil

www.ingramcontent.com/pod-product-compliance
Lightning Source LLC
Chambersburg PA
CBHW071359290426
44108CB00014B/1613